BLUE WATER NAVY VIETNAM VETERANS AND AGENT ORANGE EXPOSURE

Committee on Blue Water Navy Vietnam Veterans and Agent Orange Exposure

Board on the Health of Select Populations

INSTITUTE OF MEDICINE
OF THE NATIONAL ACADEMIES

THE NATIONAL ACADEMIES PRESS
Washington, D.C.
www.nap.edu

THE NATIONAL ACADEMIES PRESS 500 Fifth Street, N.W. Washington, DC 20001

NOTICE: The project that is the subject of this report was approved by the Governing Board of the National Research Council, whose members are drawn from the councils of the National Academy of Sciences, the National Academy of Engineering, and the Institute of Medicine. The members of the committee responsible for the report were chosen for their special competences and with regard for appropriate balance.

This study was supported by Contract V101 (93) P-2136 (Task Order 21) between the National Academy of Sciences and the Department of Veterans Affairs. Any opinions, findings, conclusions, or recommendations expressed in this publication are those of the authors and do not necessarily reflect the view of the organizations or agencies that provided support for this project.

International Standard Book Number-13: 978-0-309-16247-0
International Standard Book Number-10: 0-309-16247-5

Additional copies of this report are available from the National Academies Press, 500 Fifth Street, N.W., Lockbox 285, Washington, DC 20055; (800) 624-6242 or (202) 334-3313 (in the Washington metropolitan area); Internet, http://www.nap.edu.

For more information about the Institute of Medicine, visit the IOM home page at **www.iom.edu.**

Printed in the United States of America

The serpent has been a symbol of long life, healing, and knowledge among almost all cultures and religions since the beginning of recorded history. The serpent adopted as a logotype by the Institute of Medicine is a relief carving from ancient Greece, now held by the Staatliche Museen in Berlin.

IOM (Institute of Medicine). 2011. *Blue Water Navy Vietnam Veterans and Agent Orange Exposure.* Washington, DC: The National Academies Press.

THE NATIONAL ACADEMIES

Advisers to the Nation on Science, Engineering, and Medicine

The **National Academy of Sciences** is a private, nonprofit, self-perpetuating society of distinguished scholars engaged in scientific and engineering research, dedicated to the furtherance of science and technology and to their use for the general welfare. Upon the authority of the charter granted to it by the Congress in 1863, the Academy has a mandate that requires it to advise the federal government on scientific and technical matters. Dr. Ralph J. Cicerone is president of the National Academy of Sciences.

The **National Academy of Engineering** was established in 1964, under the charter of the National Academy of Sciences, as a parallel organization of outstanding engineers. It is autonomous in its administration and in the selection of its members, sharing with the National Academy of Sciences the responsibility for advising the federal government. The National Academy of Engineering also sponsors engineering programs aimed at meeting national needs, encourages education and research, and recognizes the superior achievements of engineers. Dr. Charles M. Vest is president of the National Academy of Engineering.

The **Institute of Medicine** was established in 1970 by the National Academy of Sciences to secure the services of eminent members of appropriate professions in the examination of policy matters pertaining to the health of the public. The Institute acts under the responsibility given to the National Academy of Sciences by its congressional charter to be an adviser to the federal government and, upon its own initiative, to identify issues of medical care, research, and education. Dr. Harvey V. Fineberg is president of the Institute of Medicine.

The **National Research Council** was organized by the National Academy of Sciences in 1916 to associate the broad community of science and technology with the Academy's purposes of furthering knowledge and advising the federal government. Functioning in accordance with general policies determined by the Academy, the Council has become the principal operating agency of both the National Academy of Sciences and the National Academy of Engineering in providing services to the government, the public, and the scientific and engineering communities. The Council is administered jointly by both Academies and the Institute of Medicine. Dr. Ralph J. Cicerone and Dr. Charles M. Vest are chair and vice chair, respectively, of the National Research Council.

www.national-academies.org

COMMITTEE ON BLUE WATER NAVY VIETNAM VETERANS AND AGENT ORANGE EXPOSURE

ROBERTA B. NESS, M.D. (*Chair*), Dean, School of Public Health, University of Texas

PATRICK N. BREYSSE, Ph.D., Professor, Department of Environmental Sciences, Johns Hopkins University Bloomberg School of Public Health

RICHARD CLAPP, D.Sc., Professor, Department of Environmental Health, Boston University

MIRIAM DIAMOND, Ph.D., Professor, Department of Geography and Program in Planning and Department of Chemical Engineering and Applied Chemistry, Dalla Lana School of Public Health, University of Toronto

MENACHEM ELIMELECH, Ph.D., Chair, Department of Chemical Engineering, Yale University

KIMBERLY L. JONES, Ph.D., Professor and Chair, Department of Civil Engineering, Howard University

SAMUEL KACEW, Ph.D., Professor of Pharmacology, McLaughlin Centre for Population Health and Risk Assessment, University of Ottawa

DAVID KALMAN, Ph.D., Chairman and Professor, Department of Environmental and Occupational Health Sciences, University of Washington

JUDY LAKIND, Ph.D., President, LaKind Associates, Associate Professor, Department of Epidemiology and Public Health, University of Maryland School of Medicine, and Adjunct Associate Professor, Department of Pediatrics, Pennsylvania State University College of Medicine, Milton S. Hershey Medical Center

JOSE SERICANO, Ph.D., Research Scientist, Geochemical and Environmental Research Group, Texas A&M University

KENNETH R. STILL, Ph.D., Director and Toxicology Consultant, Occupational Toxicology Associates Inc., and Professor, Environmental Health, School of Community Health, Portland State University

Study Staff

ROBERTA WEDGE, Study Director
MARGOT IVERSON, Program Officer
DOMINIC BROSE, Associate Program Officer
CARY HAVER, Associate Program Officer
JOSEPH GOODMAN, Senior Project Assistant
JONATHAN SCHMELZER, Senior Project Assistant
NORMAN GROSSBLATT, Senior Editor
CHRISTIE BELL, Financial Officer
RICK ERDTMANN, Director, Board on the Health of Select Populations

REVIEWERS

This report has been reviewed in draft form by persons chosen for their diverse perspectives and technical expertise in accordance with procedures approved by the National Research Council's (NRC's) Report Review Committee. The purpose of this independent review is to provide candid and critical comments that will assist the institution in making its published report as sound as possible and to ensure that the report meets institutional standards of objectivity, evidence, and responsiveness to the study charge. The review comments and draft manuscript remain confidential to protect the integrity of the deliberative process. We wish to thank the following individuals for their review of the report:

YORAM COHEN, Ph.D., University of California, Los Angeles
SEYMOUR DEITCHMAN, Independent Consultant
MICHAEL GALLO, M.D., UMDNJ–Robert Wood Johnson Medical School
DAVID H. GARABRANT, M.D., University of Michigan
ROBERT HERRICK, S.D., Harvard School of Public Health
WILLIAM LUTTRELL, Ph.D., Oklahoma Christian University
JOEL MICHALEK, Ph.D., University of Texas Health Science Center
CLAUDIA S. MILLER, M.D., University of Texas Health Science Center at San Antonio
DAVID RICHARDSON, Ph.D., University of North Carolina
THOMAS J. SMITH, Ph.D., Harvard University
RICHARD WANG, Ph.D., Centers for Disease Control and Prevention

Although the reviewers listed above have provided many constructive comments and suggestions, they were not asked to endorse the conclusions or recommendations, nor did they see the final draft of the report before its release. The review of the report was overseen by **Rogene Henderson, Ph.D.,** Lovelace Respiratory Research Institute, and **Kristine M. Gebbie, Dr.P.H., R.N.,** Flinders University of South Australia. Appointed by the NRC and the Institute of Medicine, they were responsible for making certain that an independent examination of the report was carried out in accordance with institutional procedures and that all review comments were carefully considered. Responsibility for the final content of the report rests entirely with the author committee and the institution.

PREFACE

The committee has been asked to consider whether Blue Water Navy veterans might have been exposed to herbicides used in Vietnam, specifically Agent Orange and its contaminant, 2,3,7,8-tetrachloro-dibenzo-p-dioxin (TCDD), and whether this exposure could lead to an increased risk of long-term adverse health outcomes.

When Congress passed the Agent Orange Act of 1991 (Public Law 102-4), which provided for presumption of service connections for diseases associated with exposure to certain herbicide agents, initially the law was interpreted to apply to all service men and women deployed to Vietnam including members of the Blue Water Navy. But in 2002, the Department of Veterans Affairs (VA) took the position that for a Vietnam veteran to be presumed to have been exposed to Agent Orange, the veteran must demonstrate that he or she actually set foot in Vietnam, and in 2008, that VA position was upheld by the US Court of Appeals for the Federal Circuit. This position effectively excluded most Blue Water Navy veterans from receiving a presumption of service connection for diseases associated with exposure to herbicides.

Nevertheless, Blue Water Navy Vietnam veterans continue to have concerns that they were exposed to Agent Orange and TCDD during their wartime service. A 2002 Australian study showing that TCDD could be enriched in a simulation of the distillation process used on the US Navy and Royal Australian Navy ships during the Vietnam War era to produce potable water raised awareness among Blue Water Navy veterans that a unique mechanism might exist by which they might have been exposed to TCDD. These concerns and a 2009 Institute of Medicine (IOM) *Veterans and Agent Orange* report that supported the findings of the Australian study prompted VA to ask the IOM to establish a committee to specifically study whether the Vietnam veterans in the Blue Water Navy experienced exposures to herbicides and their contaminants comparable with those of veterans who served on the inland waters of Vietnam (the Brown Water Navy) and those who served on the ground in Vietnam.

In approaching its task, the committee attempted to collect as much scientific and historical information as possible to shed light on the question of possible herbicide exposure by Blue Water Navy veterans. The committee was surprised and disheartened to find a dearth of information on environmental concentrations of TCDD during the Vietnam War, in spite of the large volumes of Agent Orange sprayed throughout South Vietnam. Such information is vital to determining possible exposures not only of Navy veterans but also veterans who served on the ground and on the inland waterways of Vietnam.

The committee struggled with how to deal with the lack of scientific data on which to base its conclusions. Because of the paucity of data available, the committee decided that it would be necessary to approach its task by evaluating whether Blue Water Navy personnel were or were not exposed to Agent Orange and its associated TCDD, and whether it is possible to state with certainty that exposure of Blue Water Navy personnel, taken as a group, was qualitatively different from that of their Brown Water Navy and ground counterparts.

Despite this limited framework for asking the question, the committee could not find enough data to determine whether or not Blue Water Navy personnel were exposed to Agent Orange–associated TCDD. At the same time, the committee could not clearly delineate whether there were overlapping exposures between personnel categories. Indeed the committee believes that given the lack of measurements taken during the war and the almost 40 years since the war, this will never be a matter of science but instead a matter of policy.

The committee appreciates the importance of this issue for many Blue Water Navy Vietnam veterans, and the committee owes a tremendous thanks to the many individuals and groups who generously gave of their time and expertise to share with committee members their insight into particular issues, to provide copies of reports and research articles, and to answer queries about their work and experiences during the war. The committee is especially grateful to the many veterans who shared their personal stories and who provided historical documents. Among the many people who provided helpful information to the committee are David Barrans, Victoria Cassano, Michael Peterson, and James Sampsel of the Department of Veterans Affairs; Susan Belanger; Thomas Boivin, Hatfield Consultants; Joseph Carnevale, US Navy (retired); Michael Cassady, US Navy; William G. Jeff Davis and Michael Teaney, Veterans Association of Sailors of the Vietnam War; Frederick Gersh; Charles Gordon, Mac McLaughlin, and the docents of the *USS Midway*; Thomas Hamrick, US Navy (retired); Clint Hoffmann, US Department of Agriculture; Mary Ellen McCarthy, Committee on Veterans' Affairs, US Senate; Paul McCarthy, US Navy (retired); John

Paul Rossie, Blue Water Navy Vietnam Veterans Association; Jeanne Stellman, Columbia University; and John Wells, US Navy (retired).

The committee is also very grateful to Roberta Wedge, who served as study director for this project, and to all of the IOM staff members who contributed to this project: Dominic Brose, Joseph Goodman, Cary Haver, Margot Iverson, and Jonathan Schmelzer. A thank you is also extended to William McLeod who conducted database and literature searches.

Roberta B. Ness, *Chair*
Committee on Blue Water Navy Vietnam Veterans and Agent Orange Exposure

CONTENTS

Tables, Figures, and Box

SUMMARY

Since the end of the Vietnam War, veterans have reported numerous health effects. Herbicides used in Vietnam, in particular Agent Orange, that contained the highly toxic chemical 2,3,7,8-tetrachloro-dibenzo-p-dioxin (also referred to as TCDD), have been associated with a variety of cancers and other long-term health effects. The Agent Orange Act of 1991 established a presumption of herbicide exposure for veterans who served in Vietnam and who developed one or more of the diseases associated with Agent Orange exposure. Such a presumption is necessary for a Vietnam veteran to receive disability compensation if he or she has an Agent Orange-associated disease. On the basis of the Institute of Medicine's (IOM's) *Veterans and Agent Orange* (*VAO*) reports and other information, the Department of Veterans Affairs (VA) has recognized the following 14 health effects as being associated with Agent Orange and other herbicide exposure: acute and subacute peripheral neuropathy, multiple myeloma, AL amyloidosis, non-Hodgkin's lymphoma (NHL), chloracne, Parkinson's disease, chronic B-cell leukemias, porphyria cutanea tarda, diabetes mellitus (type 2), prostate cancer, Hodgkin's disease, respiratory cancers, ischemic heart disease, and soft-tissue sarcoma.

Before 1997, Vietnam veterans were eligible for a presumption of exposure if "during active military, naval, or air service, they had served in the Republic of Vietnam" unless there was evidence that they had not been exposed to Agent Orange. That broad policy was later narrowed so that service on the ground in Vietnam (ground troops) or on its inland waterways (Brown Water Navy) was required to receive a presumption of exposure. The VA further stipulated that "mere service on a deep-water naval vessel in waters off shore of the Republic of Vietnam is not qualifying service in Vietnam." Those who served aboard deep-water naval vessels are the Blue Water Navy. Although that interpretation was challenged by Blue Water Navy veterans, the VA position was upheld in the 2008 case of *Haas v. Peake* and stands today. Since 2008, the VA has, case by case, recognized numerous Blue Water Navy ships as having entered the inland waterways of Vietnam or having docked in Vietnam at specific times and locations. Navy personnel who served aboard those blue-water ships during the specific times when their ships were in inland waters or docked are now eligible for the presumption of service connection for Agent Orange–associated diseases.

Blue Water Navy Vietnam veterans along with other Vietnam veterans have become concerned about their potential exposure to the TCDD contaminant present in Agent Orange. Recent publications, such as that of an Australian study of potential TCDD enrichment of potable water aboard Royal Australian Navy ships as a result of the water-distillation process, have prompted additional concerns regarding exposure of Blue Water Navy veterans to TCDD.

CHARGE TO THE COMMITTEE

The growing concern of Blue Water Navy veterans that they were exposed to Agent Orange during their service in the Vietnam War prompted the VA to task the IOM with establishing a committee to study whether the Vietnam veterans in the Blue Water Navy experienced exposures to herbicides and their contaminants comparable with those of the Brown Water Navy Vietnam veterans and those on the ground in Vietnam. The focus was to be on Agent Orange and TCDD exposures. The VA asked that the report include historical background on the Vietnam War, Agent Orange legislation, and the three veteran categories (ground troops, Brown Water Navy personnel, and Blue Water Navy personnel); a comparison of possible routes of exposure of Blue Water Navy veterans on ships and of ground troops in Vietnam, and the potential mechanisms of herbicide exposures (such as water exposure from contamination of potable water, air exposure from spray drift, and food and soil contamination); a comparison of the risks of long-term adverse health effects in ground troop veterans, Blue Water Navy veterans, and other "era" veterans who served during the Vietnam War at other locations in light of possible TCDD exposure; and a review of studies of Blue Water Navy veterans for adverse health effects (if there have been studies of that specific cohort of veterans).

COMMITTEE'S APPROACH

At the heart of this report is the question of whether Blue Water Navy veterans had the potential for exposure to the tactical herbicides used in Vietnam, specifically Agent Orange, and particularly the TCDD contaminant of that herbicide, and whether that exposure, if any, could lead to an increased risk of long-term adverse health effects. The committee's approach was to ask

- Whether it is possible to demonstrate that Blue Water Navy personnel were or were not exposed to Agent Orange–associated TCDD, and
- Whether it is possible to state with certainty that exposure of Blue Water Navy personnel, taken as a group, was qualitatively different from that of their Brown Water Navy and ground troop counterparts.

Conceptual Approach

The committee considered that the most appropriate approach for assessing the risks of long-term adverse health effects would be a risk-assessment framework. The framework begins with identifying the sources of Agent Orange and its TCDD contaminant and potential receptors (in this case, ground troops and Brown Water Navy and Blue Water Navy populations). The next step is to evaluate how Agent Orange could reach the receptors (for example, transport by soil, water, and air) and plausible routes of exposure (inhalation, dermal contact, and ingestion). The information on routes of exposure can be used in conjunction with toxicologic information to assess the health effects that TCDD may have on the receptors.

The committee began by gathering information on how Agent Orange had been used in Vietnam and the quantity and geographic range of its application. The committee also considered data on the magnitude of TCDD contamination of Agent Orange. After reviewing information on releases of Agent Orange to the environment, the committee explored the fate and transport of Agent Orange and TCDD in air, fresh and marine water, sediment, soil, and food to assess the plausibility of Agent Orange and TCDD exposure of those military personnel that did not actually handle the herbicide themselves. The committee attempted to identify any monitoring data on TCDD that had been gathered during or shortly after the Vietnam War. The committee also considered fate and transport models that could be used in conjunction with the limited available data to examine the plausibility of exposure of ground troops and Blue Water Navy veterans to the chemicals. The committee attempted to determine where Blue Water Navy ships were during the war, their missions, how close they came to the Vietnamese coast, and the activities conducted aboard the ships by the sailors in performance of their duties and during their leisure time.

To determine whether Blue Water Navy personnel had exposures to TCDD comparable with those of ground troops and Brown Water Navy personnel, the committee sought to determine whether there were plausible exposure pathways between releases of Agent Orange and TCDD (specifically, the spraying of Agent Orange during the Operation Ranch Hand missions) and the three populations.

The long-term adverse health effects of Agent Orange and TCDD have been examined by other IOM committees, particularly the VAO committees, and by other organizations, such as the International Agency for Research on Cancer. For this reason, the present committee did not review all the primary literature related to TCDD exposure and health effects, such as studies of occupational cohorts and toxicological studies with laboratory animals. Rather, it focused its literature searches and other efforts on identifying epidemiologic studies of health effects seen in Vietnam veterans that included Navy personnel as a specific population and studies that divided Navy personnel into those who may have served in the Blue Water Navy, in the Brown Water Navy, or onshore.

Information Sources

Many data sources and methods were identified and pursued by the committee, including published peer-reviewed literature, models for assessing the environmental concentrations of Agent Orange and TCDD, anecdotal information from veterans and other interested parties on veteran experiences during the war and afterwards, and such other information sources as written and published accounts of the war (including memoirs), government documents, and ships' deck logs. Although much of the information reviewed by the committee was not new, some fresh sources and documents were identified, including new VA policies, Blue Water Navy veterans' reports, materials specific to the operations of the Blue Water Navy, and further documentation of the use of Agent Orange in Vietnam.

The committee recognized the need to hold open sessions to hear directly from veterans about their experiences with Agent Orange while they served in the Vietnam War. In addition, it was agreed that much of the information that the committee would need to complete its task was not available in the published literature and that veterans would be able to provide critical information. The committee held three open sessions to collect veterans' input. At the first two sessions, held in Washington, DC, the committee heard from the VA, several veterans service organizations (for example, the Blue Water Navy Vietnam Veterans Association), numerous individual veterans, and other interested parties. The third open session was held aboard the *USS Midway*, an aircraft carrier that is now a museum, so the committee could view firsthand the distillation plants used aboard a Vietnam-era ship. Committee members found all that information to be useful in framing their approach to the committee's task and appreciating life aboard Blue Water Navy ships during the war. The committee talked with veterans of all ranks and experiences, from vice admirals to enlisted men.

Numerous other information sources also proved useful to the committee. Many of them were government documents from the VA and the Navy; other Navy documents, such as deck logs and maps; and reports from the Australian government about Australian Vietnam veterans. Several Web sites also provided useful compendiums of information, such as the site maintained by the Blue Water Navy Vietnam Veterans Association (http://www.bluewaternavy.org/) and the Virtual Vietnam Archive at Texas Tech University. Other sources of information included peer-reviewed literature and interviews with retired Navy personnel.

HISTORICAL BACKGROUND

The US government commissioned a series of studies in the middle to late 1960s evaluating possible health risks for American troops and the Vietnamese population exposed to Agent Orange. On the basis of those studies, in October 1969 the United States began limiting its use of herbicides in Vietnam; spraying ceased entirely in 1971. Additional concerns about the health dangers posed to Vietnam veterans arose after the war.

Beginning in 1979, Congress enacted several laws to determine whether exposures to herbicides in Vietnam were associated with possible long-term health effects. In 1991, Public Law (PL) 102-4, the Agent Orange Act, was passed. It required the VA to ask the IOM to conduct periodic reviews of the available scientific and medical evidence of health effects that followed exposure to herbicides used in Vietnam, including Agent Orange and its contaminant TCDD; there is currently evidence of an association between 14 health effects and exposure to Agent Orange.

Two IOM committees assessed an exposure-opportunity model developed by Columbia University principal investigator Jeanne Stellman. The model assigned an exposure-opportunity index value to individuals or groups that had homogeneous exposure characteristics (location and time); the index value was based on proximity to flight paths of aerial herbicide spraying missions and time concordance between spraying and presence in the affected areas. Full application of the exposure-opportunity model to ground troops in Vietnam was never accomplished and has never been proposed for Brown Water Navy or Blue Water Navy personnel. Although other investigators have identified differences in predicted ground-level spray deposition in the Stellman model compared with established pesticide-spray drift models such as AgDRIFT, and noted the lack of certainty in troop-location data, no alternatives to the Stellman exposure-opportunity model have been proposed.

Because of the impossibility that most Vietnam veterans could prove that they had been exposed to Agent Orange or other herbicides in Vietnam during the war, the 1991 Agent Orange Act created a presumption of service connection; that is, exposure to herbicides in Vietnam was presumed for any Vietnam veteran who became ill with a disease found to be associated with TCDD exposure. That presumption—a mechanism of disability compensation that the VA has used in other contexts—allows veterans to receive disability compensation and treatment for a medical condition without having to provide proof that the condition was "incurred in or aggravated by" their military service.

The VA denies Blue Water Navy Vietnam veterans presumptions of service connections for herbicide-related conditions unless a veteran was aboard a ship at the time of docking in Vietnam or, if shore docking did not occur, the evidence shows that the ship operated in Vietnam's close coastal waters for extended periods, members of the crew went ashore, or smaller vessels went ashore regularly from the ship with supplies or personnel. However, a ship that was in a deep-water harbor, for example,

Da Nang, would not count as being in "brown water." The VA continues to develop a list of blue-water ships documented to have entered inland waters and the dates on which they did so. Underlying the controversy of Blue Water Navy Vietnam veterans' claims to a presumption of herbicide exposure are the legal mandates to compensate veterans for their current health problems. Vietnam veterans who served on the ground and on the inland waterways of Vietnam are eligible for compensation for their Agent Orange–associated medical problems regardless of the time they spent in Vietnam and the potential for their exposure to Agent Orange during the war.

SELECTED CHEMICALS USED DURING THE VIETNAM WAR

By far the most widely used herbicide in Vietnam was Agent Orange, followed by Agent White; other tactical herbicides that were used during the war include Agent Blue, Agent Purple, Agent Pink, and Agent Green. Of the herbicides used in Vietnam, only those containing 2,4,5-trichlorophenoxyacetic acid (2,4,5-T) were contaminated with TCDD. Agent Orange was composed of equal parts 2,4,5-T and 2,4-dichlorophenoxyacetic acid as the active ingredients. TCDD occurred as a contaminant in 2,4,5-T and was present in Agent Orange at concentrations from 6.2 to 14.3 ppm (average, 13.25 ppm). It has been estimated that about 43 million liters of Agent Orange were used in Vietnam during 1965–1970. Agent Orange was applied to broad swaths of land in Vietnam, primarily via specially modified US Air Force C-123 fixed-wing aircraft during Operation Ranch Hand. A small proportion of the herbicide was also applied by other means, such as backpack sprayers, spray trucks, helicopters, and boats by the US Army Chemical Corps. An additional route of herbicide application was direct spraying of riverbanks by the Brown Water Navy.

Vietnam veterans were also exposed to other chemicals during the war. For example, in an effort to control the incidence of malaria in US ground troops in Vietnam, in 1967, the military initiated Operation Flyswatter and used modified Ranch Hand C-123 aircraft, also known as Bug Birds, to spray malathion. Unlike the C-123s used for herbicide spraying, the Bug Birds flew alone without escort aircraft and were not camouflaged. Malathion was sprayed over nine major US bases and adjacent sites every 11–14 days. Environmental conditions were similar to those used for herbicide spraying—maximum winds of 10 knots, maximum temperature of 30°C, and no rainfall during or for 1 hour after spraying.

Blue Water Navy and Brown Water Navy personnel were also exposed during the Vietnam War to many chemicals needed to operate and maintain their ships. Exposure may have occurred by ingestion, inhalation, dermal contact, or a combination of these routes. Exposure opportunity varied greatly with a sailor's occupation, the class of ship, and the nature of the activity that required the chemical (for example, painting a ship). Many of the chemicals used aboard are known to be toxic and have been demonstrated to elicit both short-term and long-term adverse health effects. The committee found it important to identify and describe some of the chemicals, their uses, and their health effects. Chemicals used aboard naval ships included solvents, jet fuel, polychlorinated biphenyls, asbestos, trichloroethylene, lead, and mercury. The committee also notes that many naval personnel smoked aboard ships with the potential for exposure to numerous toxic chemicals in cigarette smoke and exposure to secondhand smoke for nonsmokers.

Shipboard environments are influenced by ventilation systems that run throughout the entire ship. The systems have the potential to spread airborne materials collected at one site to other sites if not properly designed and maintained. The potential spread of occupationally produced airborne materials could have a serious influence on the health of shipboard personnel.

FATE AND TRANSPORT OF AGENT ORANGE AND TCDD IN THE VIETNAMESE ENVIRONMENT

Potential exposure of Blue Water Navy personnel to Agent Orange and its contaminant TCDD is related to the fate of these chemicals in the Vietnamese environment. The committee considered using a mathematical model to estimate likely TCDD concentrations based on Agent Orange inputs to the environment. All models require a host of input parameter values such as standard physical-chemical properties of TCDD, characteristics of the Vietnamese environment, and chemical- and environment-specific parameter values such as rates of TCDD degradation in the Vietnamese environment and seasonally and spatially specific knowledge of air and water movement. The committee found that input data and, importantly, data with which to evaluate model performance, were not available. Furthermore, tremendous uncertainty would accompany any attempt to model overall TCDD fate by scaling up from modeling emissions from individual spray paths for which data are available, to estimate TCDD concentrations along hundreds of miles of coastline and in coastal waters. Thus, the committee concluded that using models to estimate likely concentrations of TCDD in the Vietnamese environment to which Blue Water Navy personnel might be exposed would not be possible because of the lack of data with which to parameterize the model. Even if a model could be parameterized, data are not available to evaluate model performance. Without evaluating the model, the uncertainty of model results would be far too great and thus, the committee could not be confident that such results were reasonable.

The committee explored the variability and uncertainty of many of the input parameters that would be needed for assessing the fate and transport of TCDD in the Vietnamese environment. The goal of this exercise was to assess qualitatively the fate of TCDD released during the Vietnam War. The discussion acknowledges the importance of location-specific factors that mediate the chemical fate and transport, notably the tropical climate and geography of Vietnam. Since most of the literature on chemical fate of dioxins originates from temperate areas such as Europe and North America that differ significantly from the Vietnamese environment, the committee was mindful of these differences as its understanding of the fate TCDD in Vietnam was developed.

It has been estimated that 87% of the Agent Orange sprayed in Vietnam reached the forest canopy, while the remaining 13% drifted and was subject to atmospheric transport or degradation processes. The committee assumed that Agent Orange that did not reach the forest canopy or soils could enter the water either by direct spraying over waterways or deposition of spray drift or indirectly via land runoff.

The committee concluded that Agent Orange and TCDD would have entered waterways from riverbank spraying (although this was a small fraction of the total Agent Orange applied in Vietnam) or as runoff from soil, particularly in the Mekong delta area that was heavily sprayed and that experienced frequent flooding. This river loading would be highly diluted by river flows. A considerable fraction of particles and humic material to which TCDD would absorb, would be expected to have settled in the delta region or estuaries.

TCDD would enter the coastal marine water from river discharge and spray drift. The contribution of TCDD to marine waters from these transport routes would be reduced to a great extent by two main processes: dilution in river water and dispersion in air, as well as by further dilution in the coastal waters. Given the paucity of monitoring information and the variability and uncertainty in the fate and transport information on TCDD as it pertains to Vietnam, the committee concluded that it is not possible to estimate the likely concentrations of TCDD in marine waters and air at the time of Blue Water Navy deployment.

EXPOSURE ROUTES AND MECHANISMS

The committee was tasked with comparing exposure among three military populations that served in Vietnam: troops on the ground, Brown Water Navy personnel, and Blue Water Navy personnel. The approach used by the committee to address the task of comparing exposure among the three populations was to evaluate possible pathways of exposure of each of the three populations (termed exposure opportunities) and to consider whether it is plausible that people in these groups could have been exposed, via these pathways, to Agent Orange–associated TCDD.

The committee determined that any assessment of exposure must be qualitative rather than quantitative. Qualitative estimates should be informed by knowledge of the fate and transport of the chemicals of interest and by documented or anecdotal information on potential pathways of exposure.

The committee recognized that in addition to possible differences in exposure potential among populations, there are differences among individuals. Even ground troops or Navy personnel with similar job descriptions would be expected to have experienced varied exposure because of differences in environmental concentrations, personal activities, and associated intake characteristics (such as exposure duration, food and water ingestion rates, inhalation rate, and body weight). The committee recognizes that there may be individuals in a given group whose experiences do not accord with the descriptions given in this report. It should be noted that ground troops and Brown and Blue Water Navy personnel also included an unknown fraction of personnel who were remote from spraying operations and possibly had no opportunity for exposure.

The committee identified several plausible exposure pathways and routes of exposure to Agent Orange–associated TCDD in the three populations. Plausible pathways and routes of exposure of Blue Water

Navy personnel to Agent Orange–associated TCDD include inhalation and dermal contact with aerosols from spraying operations that occurred at or near the coast when Blue Water Navy ships were nearby, contact with marine water, and uses of potable water prepared from distilled marine water.

Large US Navy ships—such as aircraft carriers, cruisers, and destroyers—had their own potable-water supply and distribution systems that included water-treatment processes. Potable water is produced by distillation of marine water. Although the committee was told that Blue Water Navy ships did not typically make potable water within 12 miles of shore, the committee was also told that in exceptional circumstances a ship might take up water for distillation while relatively close to the coastline. The issue of distillation of marine water is important because of the finding by the committee that prepared the 2008 *VAO* update that Blue Water Navy veterans could have been exposed to TCDD via contaminated potable water. The Australian Department of Veterans Affairs determined that Royal Australian Navy personnel who served offshore were exposed to Agent Orange–associated TCDD in Vietnam because the distillation systems aboard the ships were thought to be able to concentrate TCDD in source water into the potable water during the evaporative process. This committee used a theoretical model to corroborate the findings of the experimental Australian study that found substantial codistillation of TCDD during production of potable water with a batch distillation unit that was commonly used in Blue Water Navy vessels. If Agent Orange–associated TCDD was present in the marine water, distilled potable water would be a plausible pathway of exposure.

LONG-TERM ADVERSE HEALTH EFFECTS

The long-term adverse health effects associated with exposure to dioxins have been studied in a variety of populations, including Vietnam veterans. The biennial IOM *VAO* reports have reviewed epidemiologic studies of Vietnam veterans, occupational studies, and population studies in an effort to determine whether Vietnam veterans are at increased risk for adverse health effects from exposure to Agent Orange during the Vietnam War. A few of the studies include veterans who served in the Blue Water Navy in Vietnam, but most of the studies do not distinguish

Navy veterans, let alone Blue Water Navy veterans, from other Vietnam-veteran populations.

In addition to reviewing previous *VAO* reports, the committee heard from a number of veterans and is aware that many veterans attribute their current illnesses to exposure to Agent Orange in Vietnam. The committee valued these accounts for descriptive purposes but did not have a way to use that information in its study because without a relevant control population to demonstrate that the veterans' diseases are attributable to Agent Orange–associated TCDD exposure and not other factors, the exact causes of their illnesses cannot be determined.

For Navy veterans as a whole, the Australian cancer-incidence study indicated a significantly higher risk of lung cancer (although the study did not adjust for smoking) and prostatic cancer, both of which are currently recognized as TCDD-related malignancies. The Australian study also found significant associations with melanoma and colon cancer, neither of which has been categorized as TCDD-related by the IOM or the VA. The Australian mortality study corroborated the Australian cancer-incidence findings on lung cancer and melanoma. However, both Australian reports found significantly lower risk of NHL, one of the first cancers the IOM found to be associated with Agent Orange exposure. One study found neither higher nor lower risk of NHL in Vietnam-era Navy veterans. In contrast, the Centers for Disease Control and Prevention Selected Cancers Study found a significantly higher prevalence of NHL in US Blue Water Navy Vietnam veterans. Finally, in a small study, testicular cancer was associated with service in the Navy (although the Blue Water Navy was not specified) in Vietnam veterans, although testicular cancer has not been found by the IOM to be associated with Agent Orange exposure.

Overall, the committee concludes that because of the small number of studies and their limitations, there is no consistent evidence to suggest that Blue Water Navy Vietnam veterans were at higher *or* lower risk for cancer or other long-term adverse health effects associated with Agent Orange exposure than shore-based veterans, Brown Water Navy veterans, or Vietnam veterans in other branches of service.

CONCLUSIONS

Since the 1970s, IOM committees and other groups have attempted to reconstruct Vietnam veterans' potential exposure to Agent Orange and

TCDD. Given the lack of exposure data on ground troops and the limited knowledge about exposure among Blue Water Navy veterans, the committee concluded that it was not possible to make quantitative exposure comparisons among the three military populations of interest to the VA. Therefore, the committee evaluated the *plausibility* of exposure of the three populations to Agent Orange and TCDD via various mechanisms and routes.

The committee recognized that considerable variability exists in the potential for TCDD exposure by Blue Water Navy personnel, ground troops, and Brown Water Navy personnel. Focusing on the Blue Water Navy, some personnel may have spent their entire tour of duty on aircraft carriers that never came close to the Vietnamese coast, whereas others served on ships that may have spent many days as close as 1 mile offshore. In addition to the variability in the location of Blue Water Navy personnel, there is extensive uncertainty regarding the experiences of individual sailors on those ships (for example, whether they were on a ship when it was near the Vietnamese coast, whether they went swimming, and whether they ate local food from Vietnam or Vietnamese waters).

The committee concluded that, qualitatively, ground troops and Brown Water Navy veterans had more plausible pathways of exposure (that is, there was a greater number of plausible exposure mechanisms) to Agent Orange–associated TCDD than did Blue Water Navy veterans. One exposure mechanism is specific to Blue Water Navy ships: possible TCDD contamination of potable water from onboard distillation plants. The committee's assessment corroborates the Australian finding that in experiments simulating the water-distillation system used on Navy ships the system had the potential to enrich TCDD concentrations from the feed water to the distilled potable water. However, without information on the TCDD concentrations in the marine feed water, it is impossible to determine whether Blue Water Navy personnel were exposed to Agent Orange–associated TCDD via ingestion, dermal contact, or inhalation of potable water.

The committee was unable to state with certainty that Blue Water Navy personnel *were or were not* exposed to Agent Orange and its associated TCDD. Owing to a lack of data on environmental concentrations of Agent Orange and Agent Orange–associated TCDD and an inability to reconstruct likely concentrations, as well as the dearth of information about relative exposures among the ground troops and Brown Water Navy personnel and Blue Water Navy personnel, it is impossible to compare actual exposures across these three populations. Furthermore, the committee concludes that because of the small number of studies and their limitations, there is no consistent evidence to suggest that Blue Water Navy Vietnam veterans were at higher or lower risk for cancer or other long-term adverse health effects associated with Agent Orange exposure than shore-based veterans, Brown Water Navy veterans, or Vietnam veterans in other branches of service.

The committee's judgment is that exposure of Blue Water Navy Vietnam veterans to Agent Orange–associated TCDD cannot reasonably be determined.

1

INTRODUCTION

The Vietnam War era is considered by the US Department of Veterans Affairs (VA) to have lasted from January 1962 to May 1975. During that time, over 3 million US military personnel were sent to Southeast Asia. During World War II, US forces that fought in tropical climates with jungle foliage throughout the Pacific theater suffered substantial loss of lives. In the Vietnam War, the US military had new weapons to help its personnel to penetrate the tropical forests: tactical herbicides. Those herbicides were used as defoliants to help in identifying enemy transportation and communication routes and camps, to reduce cover for enemy forces, and, for a time, to kill crops that might be used by the enemy. Of the several herbicides used in Vietnam, the best known and most widely used was Agent Orange. Agent Orange was contaminated with the highly toxic chemical 2,3,7,8-tetrachlorodibenzo-p-dioxin, also referred to as TCDD.

Since that time, veterans who served in Vietnam have reported numerous adverse health effects. Beginning in 1979, Congress enacted several laws to examine links between exposures to the herbicides used in Vietnam and possible long-term health effects. In 1984, Congress required the VA to establish guidelines and standards for evaluating the scientific studies related to the exposures and to issue regulations for adjudicating claims for VA benefits based on herbicide exposure. The Agent Orange Act of 1991 established a presumption of herbicide exposure for veterans who had served in Vietnam and who developed one or more of the diseases associated with Agent Orange; an amendment in 2001 maintained the presumption of herbicide exposure but removed the need for veterans to have developed a herbicide-associated disease. On the basis of the Institute of Medicine (IOM) *Veterans and Agent Orange* (*VAO*) reports and other information, the VA has recognized 14 health outcomes as associated with Agent Orange and other herbicide exposure and thus eligible for a presumption of service connection (see Box 1-1). The 1991 legislation also asked the National Academy of Sciences, through the IOM, to conduct periodic reviews of the scientific and medical evidence connecting certain herbicide exposures to health effects. The IOM issued its first *VAO* report in 1994; the latest report, *Veterans and Agent Orange, Update 2008*, was published in 2009.

Before 1997, Vietnam veterans were eligible for a presumption of exposure to any of four herbicides used in Vietnam—2,4-dichlorophenoxyacetic acid (Agent Purple, Agent Orange, and Agent White), 2,4,5-trichlorophenoxyacetic acid (Agent Green, Agent Pink, Agent Purple, Agent Orange), cacodylic acid (Agent Blue), and picloram—if "during active military, naval, or air service, they had served in the Republic of Vietnam" unless there was evidence that they had *not* been exposed. A veteran's receipt of the Vietnam Service Medal or service in the offshore waters of Vietnam was sufficient to establish a presumption of herbicide exposure. That broad policy was later narrowed so that service on the ground in Vietnam (ground troops) or on its inland waterways (Brown Water Navy) was required to receive a presumption of exposure. Service in the Republic of Vietnam under 38 CFR § 3.307(a)(6)(iii) was defined as actual service in the country, including inland waterways, from January 9, 1962, to May 7, 1975, and service offshore if the conditions of service involved duty or visitation onshore. The VA further stipulated that "mere service on a deep-water naval vessel in waters off shore of the Republic of Vietnam is not qualifying service in Vietnam" (VA, 1997).

BOX 1-1
Veterans' Diseases Associated with Agent Orange Exposure

- Acute and subacute peripheral neuropathy
- AL amyloidosis
- Chloracne
- Chronic B-cell leukemias
- Diabetes mellitus (type 2)
- Hodgkin's disease
- Ischemic heart disease
- Multiple myeloma
- Non-Hodgkin's lymphoma
- Parkinson's disease
- Porphyria cutanea tarda
- Prostate cancer
- Respiratory cancers
- Soft-tissue sarcoma

SOURCE: See http://www.publichealth.va.gov/exposures/agentorange/diseases.asp (accessed January 19, 2011).

Those who served aboard deep-water naval vessels are the Blue Water Navy. Within the current VA interpretation, Blue Water Navy personnel are not eligible for a presumption of exposure. Although that interpretation was challenged by Blue Water Navy veterans, the VA position was upheld in the 2008 case of *Haas v. Peake* and stands today. Since 2008, the VA has, case by case, recognized numerous Blue Water Navy ships as having entered the inland waterways of Vietnam or having docked in Vietnam at specific times and locations. Navy personnel who served aboard those blue-water ships during the specific times when their ships were on inland waters or docked are now eligible for the presumption of service connection to Agent Orange–associated diseases. The VA continues to review the deck logs and other materials for Blue Water Navy ships to determine their crews' eligibility for consideration of the presumption of exposure to herbicides, but this process has been slow and labor intensive. As of January 2011, over 140 individual ships and 51 classes of Navy vessels that served in the Seventh Fleet during the Vietnam era have been categorized as having served primarily or exclusively in inland waterways, temporarily in inland waterways, or in coastal waterways of Vietnam with evidence that crew members went ashore or that smaller ships regularly went ashore with supplies or personnel (James Sampsel, VA, personal communication, January 12, 2011). Navy personnel who served aboard Blue Water Navy ships that have not been categorized as brown-water ships or who served on such ships before or after the designated period of brown water activity are not eligible for the presumption of service connection.

Blue Water Navy Vietnam veterans have been active in notifying the VA of ships that entered Vietnamese inland waters by submitting deck logs and other documentation. They have also been active in working with members of Congress to enact legislation to expand the eligibility for presumption of herbicide exposure to Blue Water Navy veterans, although such legislation has not been enacted. Their concerns are related to potential exposure not only to the herbicides themselves but to the TCDD contaminant present in Agent Orange. Recent publications, such as that of an Australian study of potential TCDD enrichment of potable water onboard Royal Australian Navy ships as a result of the ships' water-distillation process, have prompted additional concerns regarding exposure of Blue Water Navy veterans to herbicide-related TCDD (Muller et al., 2002).

The IOM committee that prepared the 2008 update in the *VAO* report series stated:

> The evidence that this committee has reviewed makes limiting *Vietnam service* [emphasis in original] to those who set foot on Vietnamese soil seem inappropriate. The ongoing series of hearings and appeals in the US Court of Appeals for Veterans Claims (*Haas v. Nicholson*) reflect the controversy.... There is little reason to believe that exposure of US military personnel to the herbicides sprayed in Vietnam was limited to those who actually set foot in the Republic of Vietnam. Having reviewed the Australian report (Muller et al., 2002) on the fate of TCDD when seawater is distilled to produce potable water, the committee is convinced that this use of seawater would provide a feasible route of exposure of personnel in the Blue Water Navy, which might have been supplemented by drift from herbicide spraying.... The present [2008] committee notes that all previous VAO committees have considered information on naval Vietnam veterans to pertain to possible Agent Orange exposure when evaluating the full spectrum of health outcomes. The present committee finds that exposure assignment to be appropriate. No new studies considered in this update contained Navy-specific information, but such information has been factored into the evolving conclusions of VAO committees. Given the available evidence, the committee recommends that members of the Blue Water Navy should not be excluded from the set of Vietnam-era veterans with presumed herbicide exposure. (IOM, 2009)

COMMITTEE'S CHARGE

The growing concern of Blue Water Navy veterans that they were exposed to Agent Orange and TCDD during their service during the Vietnam War, possibly as a result of drinking contaminated water, prompted the VA to task the IOM with establishing a committee to

> conduct a study and prepare a report on whether the Vietnam veterans in the Blue Water Navy experienced a comparable range of exposures to herbicides and their contaminants (focus on dioxin) as the Brown Water Navy Vietnam veterans and those on the ground in Vietnam (i.e., specifically with regard to

Agent Orange exposure). The IOM committee's report is expected to include

- Historical background on the Vietnam War, combat troops (ground troops), Brown Water Navy (includes inland waters), Blue Water Navy, and VAO legislation;
- A discussion of exposures (Blue Water Navy in comparison with ground troops in Vietnam), specifically, a comparison of exposures on ground with those on ships (discuss all possible routes of exposure), and examining the range of exposure mechanisms for herbicide exposures (i.e., concentrating toxics in drinking water, air exposure possibly from drift from spraying, food, soil, skin);
- A determination, if possible, of the comparative risks for long-term health outcomes comparing Vietnam veteran ground troops, Blue Water Navy veterans, and other "era" veterans serving during the Vietnam War at other locations (given the possible dioxin exposure); and
- A review of studies of Blue Water Navy veterans for health outcomes (assuming there are studies specific to that cohort of veterans).

COMMITTEE'S APPROACH TO ITS CHARGE

The committee was tasked with describing possible routes of exposure of Blue Water Navy personnel during the Vietnam War to herbicides, particularly Agent Orange, and their contaminants, specifically TCDD, and compare those exposures with ground troops in Vietnam. The committee was not tasked with nor did it attempt to determine what health effects have been associated with exposure to TCDD. Rather the committee relied on health effects assessments of TCDD made by organizations such as the US Environmental Protection Agency (EPA), and other IOM committees.

The committee describes below its conceptual approach to those tasks and the sources that it used for information on which to base its conclusions.

Conceptual Approach

At the heart of this report is the question of whether Blue Water Navy veterans had the potential for exposure to the tactical herbicides used in Vietnam, specifically Agent Orange, and particularly the TCDD contaminant of that herbicide, and whether that exposure, if any, could lead to increased risk of long-term adverse health outcomes. The committee's approach was to ask

- Whether it is possible to demonstrate that Blue Water Navy personnel were or were not exposed to Agent Orange–associated TCDD, and
- Whether it is possible to state with certainty that exposure of Blue Water Navy personnel, taken as a group, was qualitatively different from that of their Brown Water Navy and ground counterparts.

The committee considered that the most appropriate approach for assessing the risks would be the risk-assessment framework used by the EPA, albeit with modifications specific to these populations and in consideration of the available data. The framework begins with identifying the sources of the environmental agent (in this case, the herbicides used in Vietnam, particularly Agent Orange and its TCDD contaminant) and potential receptors (in this case, ground troops and Brown Water Navy and Blue Water Navy populations). The next step is to evaluate how the chemicals move in the environment to reach the populations of interest (for example, via transport in soil, water, and air) and plausible routes of exposure (inhalation, dermal contact, and ingestion). That information is used in conjunction with toxicologic information to assess the health outcomes, such as cancer, diabetes, and neurologic effects, that the chemicals may have on the populations of interest.

Given the conclusions reached by previous VAO committees, the present committee decided that the focus of its report would be on exposure to Agent Orange and not to the other tactical herbicides used in Vietnam, such as Agent Purple, Agent White, and Agent Blue. Agent Orange was used in far greater quantities and over a larger area of Vietnam than were the other herbicides. The earlier VAO committees had determined that TCDD was the most toxic substance to which

Vietnam veterans may have been exposed during their tours of duty; therefore, the present committee focused on Agent Orange and TCDD.

In the sections below, the committee describes its approach to assessing veterans' exposure to and health outcomes associated with Agent Orange and TCDD during the Vietnam War.

Sources of Agent Orange in the Environment

The committee began by gathering information on how Agent Orange and the other tactical herbicides had been used in Vietnam and the quantity and geographic range of herbicide application. The committee also considered data on the magnitude of TCDD contamination of Agent Orange. Much of that information had been collected and evaluated by earlier IOM committees and other researchers. Primary among the data available to earlier IOM committees were Department of Defense (DoD) Herbicide Reporting System records on Operation Ranch Hand, a file containing information on each Ranch Hand mission. Operation Ranch Hand was the code name for the US military's use of tactical herbicides in the Republic of Vietnam (and Laos) during the Vietnam War.

Fate and Transport of Agent Orange and TCDD in Vietnam

After reviewing information on releases of Agent Orange in the environment, the committee explored the fate and transport of TCDD in air, water, and soil to assess the plausibility of Agent Orange and TCDD exposure of military personnel that did not handle the herbicide themselves. The committee attempted to identify any monitoring data on TCDD that had been gathered during or shortly after the Vietnam War. Such monitoring data would include samples from environmental media (soil, air, water, sediment, and food) and any biologic samples collected from military personnel (such as blood samples). The committee also considered fate and transport models that could be used to examine the plausibility of exposure of ground troops, Brown Water Navy veterans, and Blue Water Navy veterans to the chemicals.

Blue Water Navy Operations and Locations

An understanding of where and how the Blue Water Navy operated was considered to be important in assessing whether veterans had any potential for exposure to Agent Orange and TCDD. Unlike the previous VAO committees, which did not distinguish among Vietnam veteran populations in terms of potential Agent Orange and TCDD exposure, the present committee was required to make such distinctions so it could discuss exposure and risks of long-term health effects specifically in Blue Water Navy veterans. Therefore, the committee attempted to identify where Blue Water Navy ships were during the war, their missions, how close they came to the Vietnamese coast, whether they docked in Vietnam, and the activities conducted aboard the ships and possibly ashore by the sailors in performance of their duties and during their leisure time. Such information would assist the committee in comparing Agent Orange and TCDD exposures potentially experienced by ground troops, Brown Water Navy veterans, and Blue Water Navy veterans. The committee also sought information that would help it to coordinate ship locations with Ranch Hand spray missions and fate and transport data on TCDD to establish what, if any, Blue Water Navy ships may have had a potential for TCDD exposure.

Routes of Exposure

One of the committee's tasks was to determine whether Blue Water Navy veterans had exposures to TCDD comparable with those of ground troops and Brown Water Navy veterans. To accomplish that task, the committee sought to determine whether there were plausible exposure pathways between the release of Agent Orange (the spraying of Agent Orange, primarily by fixed-wing aircraft, and riverbank spraying) and Blue Water Navy personnel. Therefore, the committee assessed the fate and transport of TCDD in each environmental medium as described above. On the basis of that assessment, various exposure mechanisms and routes of exposure were assessed to determine the plausibility of exposure.

Long-Term Adverse Health Outcomes

The long-term adverse health outcomes associated with exposure to TCDD have been examined by other IOM committees, particularly the VAO committees, and by other organizations, such as the EPA and the International Agency for Research on Cancer. The VAO committees identified and reviewed studies of Vietnam veterans that assessed possible health effects associated with TCDD exposure. Those studies generally used control groups of veterans who served in the armed forces during the Vietnam War but who were not deployed to Vietnam—the "Vietnam-era veterans." Given the breadth of the studies considered by those groups and the fact that the studies have previously been subjected to peer review, the present committee elected not to review the primary literature related to long-term adverse health effects that might result from TCDD exposure, such as studies of occupational cohorts and animals. Rather, it focused its literature searches and other efforts on identifying epidemiologic studies of health effects seen in Vietnam veterans that included Navy personnel as a specific study group and studies that divided Navy personnel into those who may have served in the Blue Water Navy, in the Brown Water Navy, or onshore.

Information Sources

To accomplish the tasks laid out in the conceptual approach, the committee used a multitude of data sources and methods to determine what work had been done on the exposure of Vietnam veterans to TCDD and what studies had been undertaken to assess the health effects associated with TCDD exposure. What sets the present effort apart from other efforts to assess the health of Vietnam veterans is the need to determine whether Blue Water Navy Vietnam veterans experienced different exposures and thus different health risks compared to other Vietnam veterans. That required an understanding of Blue Water Navy activities in Vietnam—from ship locations to daily activities aboard the ships or ashore during port visits. The committee also needed to be able to compare the experiences of these veterans with those of ground troops (Army soldiers and marines) and of Brown Water Navy veterans, where possible.

Many data sources and methods were identified and pursued, including published peer-reviewed literature, models for assessing the environmental concentrations of TCDD, modeling the likely transfer of TCDD from sea water to the potable water used aboard Blue Water Navy ships, and information from veterans and other interested parties on veteran experiences during the war and afterwards, and such other information sources as written and published accounts of the war (including memoirs), government documents, and ships' deck logs. Although much of the information reviewed by the committee was not new, some fresh sources and documents were identified, including new VA policies, Blue Water Navy veterans' reports, materials specific to the operations of the Blue Water Navy, and further documentation of the use of Agent Orange in Vietnam. The information sources used by the committee are discussed below.

Published Literature

Several methods were used by the committee to search for published studies of Vietnam Navy veterans and Agent Orange and TCDD exposure. The search included studies of non-American Navy veterans of the Vietnam War, such as veterans who served in the Royal Australian Navy. The first method used was a review of the biennial *VAO* IOM reports (1994–2008). The second method was an exhaustive database search. IOM library staff searched MEDLINE, EMBASE, National Technical Information Service, PsychINFO, SCOPUS, Web of Science, WorldCat, JSTOR, DTIC (Defense Technical Info Center), and Lexis Nexis databases, using search terms intended to identify any epidemiologic studies of Vietnam-era Navy personnel.

Other studies in the published literature that were retrieved included studies of the fate and transport of Agent Orange and TCDD in the environment and studies that assessed the potential exposure of Vietnam veterans to these chemicals. Although not always peer-reviewed, books that discussed those subjects were also retrieved, such as a 2009 book by Alvin Young on the use, disposition, and fate of the tactical herbicides used in the Vietnam War; veterans' memoirs and accounts of the war to help the committee to understand the day-to-day activities of the men and women who served during the war; and scholarly histories of Navy operations during the war, including books that described Navy ships and their classes and specifications.

In addition to published studies in peer-reviewed journals, the committee looked for published documents in the "gray literature." They were found through additional database searches by the IOM information specialist and Internet searches by IOM staff. Documents that were obtained in that manner included such reports as those by Hatfield Consultants on dioxin concentrations in present-day Vietnam.

Public Input

From the beginning of the committee's deliberations, open sessions were held to hear directly from veterans themselves about their experiences with Agent Orange while they served in the Vietnam War. In addition, it was agreed that much of the information that the committee would need to complete its task was not available in the published literature and that veterans would be able to provide certain types of critical information. The committee held three open sessions to collect public input. At the first and third sessions, held in Washington, DC, the committee heard from the VA, several veterans service organizations (for example, the Blue Water Navy Vietnam Veterans Association), numerous individual veterans, and other interested parties. The second open session was held aboard the *USS Midway*, an aircraft carrier that is now a museum in San Diego, so that the committee could view firsthand the distillation plants used aboard a Vietnam-era ship. Docents on the *USS Midway* explained and answered questions about the working of the plants. The committee found these information sources useful in framing its approach to its task and appreciating life aboard Blue Water Navy ships during the war. Committee members talked with veterans of many ranks and experiences, from vice admirals to enlisted men.

Several veterans provided the committee with numerous reports, articles from the peer-reviewed literature and popular press, and other documentation, all of which the committee considered during its deliberations. Veterans also talked with IOM staff about specific activities aboard Blue Water Navy ships. Finally, many veterans and their family members and friends sent e-mails to the committee; most of these e-mail messages pertained specifically to Blue Water Navy veterans' experiences during the war and their later health issues.

Other Information Sources

Numerous other information sources also proved useful to the committee. These included government documents from the VA and the Navy; other Navy documents, such as deck logs and maps; and reports from the Australian government about Australian Vietnam veterans. Several Web sites also provided useful compendiums of information, such as the site maintained by the Blue Water Navy Vietnam Veterans Association (http://www.bluewaternavy.org/) and the Virtual Vietnam Archive at Texas Tech University.

Navy documents, such as *Machinist's Mate 2 & 3*: "Steam Operated Distilling Plants," (Department of the Navy, 2003) assisted the committee in understanding the operations of the water-distillation systems that provided potable water to the crew aboard Blue Water Navy ships—a critical issue, as noted in the discussion of the committee's charge. Other Navy regulations indicated where and when such water could be prepared.

Given the committee's interest in identifying where ships were with respect to the spraying of Agent Orange, documentation to this effect was also sought. Ship logs were one source of information, but the committee was provided neither the time nor the resources to review individual deck logs to ascertain where a certain ship was at any given time; additionally, this was considered to be outside the scope of the committee's charge. However, the logs were useful in providing evidence of how far off the coast of Vietnam some ships were stationed. The difficulty in using deck logs is the need to coordinate the dates of Ranch Hand missions near the coast with the identification of ships that were near the flight paths and how far off the coast the ships were on the dates of the spraying missions. Several Web sites, such as http://www.history.navy.mil/branches/org10-8.htm and http://www.cc.gatech.edu/~tpilsch/AirOps/ranch.html, provided useful summaries of ship locations, and these were also considered by the committee.

The VA provided background information on the Blue Water Navy Vietnam veterans' issues, including a presentation to the committee on compensation and the history of the court case (*Haas v. Peake*) that resulted in Blue Water Navy Vietnam veterans no longer being presumed to have had herbicide exposure during the war. The VA is reviewing deck logs case by case to classify ships that entered inland waters as Brown Water Navy ships and would thus be eligible for the presumption of herbicide exposure. As each ship is recategorized, it is listed in the VA *Compensation and Pension Service Bulletin*. The committee received copies of the bulletin, documentation from the *Haas v. Peake* case, and a document from the Board of Veterans' Appeals lecture series on herbicide exposure (Janec and Smith, 2009).

As noted in the committee's charge and the 2008 *VAO* report, the decision by the Royal Australian Navy to compensate Australian Navy Vietnam veterans for TCDD exposure was an impetus for the current study by the IOM. The Australian decision was based on several reports that showed that Australian Navy veterans had higher incidences of some cancers than Navy veterans who had not served in Vietnam. A further Australian report suggested that TCDD may have been concentrated in the potable water of the Navy ships as a result of the water-distillation processes used on the ships. The committee thoroughly reviewed those documents and contacted the Royal Australian Navy to seek further information on the issue.

ORGANIZATION OF THE REPORT

Chapter 2 of this report provides a short historical background on the Vietnam War and the military personnel who constituted the ground combat troops, the Brown Water Navy, and the Blue Water Navy. It also presents a synopsis of the legislation regarding veterans and Agent Orange since the Vietnam War and of the recent legal issues that have arisen over Blue Water Navy veterans' compensation. In Chapter 3, the committee describes the use of tactical herbicides during the Vietnam War, particularly Agent Orange, and some of the chemicals to which naval personnel may have been exposed while on active duty. The environment of Vietnam and the fate and transport of Agent Orange–associated TCDD are explored in Chapter 4 with a discussion of the role of modeling in estimating environmental concentrations of TCDD. Chapter 5 addresses the committee's task of comparing exposure of ground troops with Navy personnel on ships and explores the mechanisms by which these military personnel may have been exposed to Agent Orange. The comparative risks of long-term health effects in ground troops, Blue Water Navy veterans, and other veterans who served during the war but were not deployed to Vietnam are presented in Chapter 6. Finally, in Chapter 7, the committee summarizes what it has learned about the potential exposure of and health effects in Blue Water Navy Vietnam veterans. An appendix reviews the Australian report *Examination of the Potential Exposure of Royal Australian Navy Personnel to Polychlorinated Dibenzodioxins and Polychlorinated Dibenzofurans via Drinking Water* (Muller et al., 2002).

REFERENCES

Department of the Navy. 2003. *Machinist's mate 3 & 2 (Surface)*. NAVEDTRA 14151. Pensacola, FL: Naval Education and Training, Professional Development and Technology Center.

IOM (Institute of Medicine). 2009. *Veterans and Agent Orange: Update 2008*. Washington, DC: The National Academies Press.

Janec, S., and T. Smith. 2009. Herbicide exposure. In *Board of Veterans' Appeals Lecture Series*. Washington, DC: Department of Veterans Affairs.

Muller, J. F., C. Gaus, K. Bundred, V. Alberts, M. R. Moore, and K. Horsley. 2002. *Examination of the potential exposure of Royal Australian Navy (RAN) personnel to polychlorinated dibenzodioxins and polychlorinated dibenzofurans via drinking water. A report to: The Department of Veteran Affairs, Australia.* Brisbane, Australia: National Research Centre for Environmental Toxicology.

VA (Department of Veterans Affairs). 1997. *Service in the Republic of Vietnam for purposes of definition of Vietnam Era—1-38 U.S.C. § 101(29)(A). Memorandum from VA General Counsel to Director of Compensation and Pension Service.* VAOPGCPREC 27-97. July 23, 1997.

2

HISTORICAL BACKGROUND

Over the last decade, a controversy has arisen regarding whether Blue Water Navy Vietnam veterans were potentially exposed to the same tactical herbicides as were their fellow veterans who served on the ground or on the inland waterways in Vietnam. This chapter presents a brief chronology of the issues surrounding the question of whether they were potentially exposed to herbicides, particularly Agent Orange and its contaminant 2,3,7,8-tetrachlorodibenzo-p-dioxin, also referred to as TCDD, and thus should be eligible for compensation. A summary of American involvement in Vietnam, focusing on the role of the Blue Water Navy, is presented first, including a discussion of the missions and roles of the several Navy sectors, such as the Brown Water Navy and the Coast Guard. A synopsis of the legislation regarding veterans and Agent Orange since the Vietnam War and of the recent legal issues that have arisen over Blue Water Navy veterans' compensation then follows.

AMERICAN INVOLVEMENT IN THE VIETNAM WAR

American involvement in Southeast Asia did not begin with the Vietnam War. After World War II, when Vietnam became an independent nation, the US government supported France's interest in repossessing Vietnam, its former colony. Its support grew primarily out of an American interest in building alliances with Western European nations that would fight against the Soviet Union's expansion efforts of the early Cold War. After the Communist victory in China in 1949 and the beginning of the Korean War in 1950, the US government expanded its financial and advisory support of the French in the French-Vietnamese conflict (also known as the First Indochina War). In 1950, the US Military Assistance Advisory Group-Indochina (MAAG-Indochina) was established, and small numbers of American military personnel went to Saigon to supervise the material support that the United States was providing to the French (Marolda, 1994).

In 1954, the Vietnamese defeated the French forces, and the two sides agreed to a temporary, 2-year partition of Vietnam at the 17th parallel, with the French military forces retreating to the south before elections were held and a unified government could be established. The US government publicly supported that plan but privately provided funding and other support for the development of an independent, anticommunist, pro-American state in the south, the Republic of Vietnam. In the late 1950s, the government of North Vietnam, the Democratic Republic of Vietnam, ratcheted up its efforts to take over South Vietnam and merge the two countries; in 1960, it established the National Liberation Front (the NLF, commonly known to Americans as the Viet Cong) to fight against the South Vietnam government (Appy, 1993; Marolda, 1994). In August 1964, shots were allegedly fired at the American destroyer *USS Maddox* off the coast of North Vietnam in the Gulf of Tonkin, where it was conducting intelligence-gathering on behalf of the Republic of Vietnam. President Lyndon Johnson ordered retaliatory air strikes on North Vietnam, and Congress later passed the Gulf of Tonkin Resolution, sending large numbers of US troops to Vietnam. US troop levels in South Vietnam rapidly rose from 23,000 ground troops in 1964 to 185,000 in 1965 and peaked in 1968 with 536,000 ground troops (Appy, 1993).

In early 1968, the "Tet Offensive" campaign by the NLF and South Vietnamese irregulars began a period of intense fighting (Turley, 2009) and helped to turn an already disillusioned American public more sharply against the war. President Johnson ordered a slow withdrawal of American troops from Vietnam. American troop withdrawal began in 1969, and the transfer of military equipment and leadership responsibilities to the South Vietnamese government (known as the Vietnamization of the war effort) became a larger focus of the American military. American troop levels decreased rapidly thereafter, and in 1973 after the Paris Peace Accord, virtually all remaining American troops were withdrawn. Fighting continued between North Vietnam and South Vietnam, however, until April 30, 1975, when Saigon, the capitol of South Vietnam, was captured by the North Vietnamese, and the South Vietnamese army surrendered.

The Blue Water Navy in the Vietnam War

The Blue Water Navy commonly refers to ships designed for open-ocean sailing and by association to the sailors assigned to those ships.

For example, the quintessential Blue Water Navy ship is the aircraft carrier, which can easily sail across an ocean but is less able to enter coastal waters (only in large deep-water ports) or to travel on inland waters. The Blue Water Navy is often juxtaposed with the Brown Water Navy, which comprises vessels that are best suited for operations very close to shore or on inland waters, such as rivers and bays, and are often not seaworthy for extended trips or for rough weather. In Vietnam, the quintessential Brown Water Navy vessels were the river patrol boat and the fast patrol boat (also known as the swift boat).

Another definition of the Blue Water Navy has developed with regard to the Vietnam War for legal purposes in determining eligibility for a presumptive service connection of diseases associated with exposure to tactical herbicides. In the present report, *blue water* refers to the more narrow legal definition of persons who served in the Navy during the Vietnam War and were stationed on ships that spent time in the waters offshore of Vietnam but never entered inland waters or set foot on land in Vietnam.

The Seventh Fleet, which is the section of the US Navy Pacific Fleet permanently stationed in the Western Pacific, had a presence in Vietnam and Vietnamese waters dating to 1950 as part of MAAG-Indochina. Navy personnel in Saigon supervised the transfer of naval supplies, including several aircraft carriers and over 400 other ships, first to the French and later to the South Vietnamese government. The Navy also provided training and advice to the nascent South Vietnamese Navy and executed shows of force of US ships in the waters surrounding North Vietnam and South Vietnam in support of the South Vietnamese government. In the early 1960s, the fleet increased; by 1965, Navy ships were involved in a wide array of blue-water and brown-water operations in and around Vietnam. At the peak of American involvement in the Vietnam War, in 1968, there were 38,000 Navy personnel in NAVFORV (Naval Forces Vietnam); this decreased to about 17,000 by the end of 1970 (Marolda, 1994).

By the end of the War, the Navy played a minimal role in near-shore and in-country activities. The Treaty of Paris limited the number of American military personnel who could be involved in any military assistance to the Republic of Vietnam, and the Navy's main contribution was to assist in the evacuation of Americans (military and civilian) and Vietnamese refugees from South Vietnam. The Navy was also involved in the evacuation of Cambodia.

American naval operations in the Vietnam War had multiple goals during the period of 1965 to 1973, but most operations can be classified as aerial bombing and surveillance, surface interdiction of supplies along the coast and inland waterways, gunfire support, logistical support, military advising, and humanitarian efforts (Marolda, 1994).

Offshore Air Operations

Aircraft carriers and their affiliated combat and support ships conducted numerous aerial bombing campaigns throughout the war. Those operations were intended both to damage enemy equipment and to affect morale. Carrier ship groups comprised a flagship aircraft carrier and multiple destroyers, cruisers, and support ships that stored ammunition, fuel, and other supplies (also referred to as carrier divisions or carrier strike groups). Carrier ship groups also participated in aerial interdiction and surveillance missions and conducted search-and-rescue missions for downed pilots. Examples of substantial carrier bombing operations include Operation Flaming Dart; Operation Rolling Thunder, which was an aerial bombing campaign over North Vietnam; and Operation Barrel Roll, which targeted Laos.

Carrier groups assigned to bombing operations would often be rotated into active bombing duties for a period of days or a month, during which a carrier group was responsible for running air bombing operations for a particular number of hours per day in one of the two major offshore operating areas used by the Navy in Vietnam (Yankee Station off northern South Vietnam and Dixie Station in the south), which were interspersed with short visits to the Subic Bay naval base in the Philippines. Carrier ship groups involved in bombing campaigns aimed at North Vietnam and Laos were often based at Yankee Station, which was about 100 miles offshore of South Vietnam due east of Dong Hoi in the Gulf of Tonkin. Carriers engaged in bombing missions over South Vietnam were also based at Dixie Station, which was about 80 miles southeast of Cam Ranh Bay in the South China Sea. Those operations did not routinely move carriers close to the Vietnam coastline.

At any given time, two to four carrier groups each were on active duty at Yankee Station and Dixie Station. Carrier crews varied in size depending on the class of the ship, but each carrier required a crew of about 3,000 to 5,500 men. Those crews were by far the largest in the fleet and thus a substantial proportion of sailors who served in the Blue Water Navy in Vietnam served aboard carriers. Destroyers carried complements of several hundred men, and cruisers generally 1,000–1,400 men.

Coastal Surface Surveillance and Interdiction

Blue Water Navy ships also patrolled the coast of South Vietnam and adjoining countries to intercept vessels attempting to smuggle troops or supplies to the enemy. Destroyers and cruisers worked with spotter planes to identify and destroy enemy vessels, and their efforts complemented the work of the smaller brown-water ships and boats that would patrol shallow waters close to shore and inland waterways.

Examples of substantial surface interdiction operations included Operation Sea Dragon (1966–1968), which operated along the coast of North Vietnam, and Operation Market Time (1965–1973), which focused on the South Vietnamese coastline. Those operations involved both Blue Water Navy and Brown Water Navy vessels.

Surface Gunfire Support

Another role of the Blue Water Navy was to supply surface gunfire support to ground troops in Vietnam. Gunfire support was provided primarily by cruisers and destroyers, which were stationed offshore within range of targets, fired for a period of hours or days, and then returned to safer locations farther offshore to reload ammunition and conduct repairs before rotating back onto the firing line. The ships often worked in teams to keep gunlines manned at all times. The committee heard from several navy veterans the gunline could be as close as one mile offshore, depending on such variables as how far inland the targets were, whether and to what extent they were experiencing enemy fire, and the range of their guns.

Logistics and Transport

Naval ships played a minor role in the transport of people and supplies from the US mainland to Vietnam. At the beginning of the war, there was some trans-Pacific troop transport on Navy ships, but most ground troops were arriving by commercial airline by the end of 1966. Navy ships did, however, transport some troops after their arrival in Vietnam. For example, amphibious transport dock ships, such as the *Duluth*, transported ground troops to the coastal waters of Vietnam; the troops would either travel to shore via smaller landing vessels or directly disembark to Vietnam if the ship docked (if the ship docked, sailors aboard at the time would be considered brown-water sailors under current VA compensation regulations; see discussion later in this chapter).

Some Navy ships were tasked primarily with providing logistical support. Many auxiliary ships—including floating barracks and floating base platforms, hospital ships, gasoline tankers, and repair ships—regularly docked in bays or traveled the inland waters in Vietnam and so are not considered part of the Blue Water Navy.

The Brown Water Navy in the Vietnam War

A primary mission of the Brown Water Navy was to prevent the movement of supplies supporting the NLF along the rivers and coastal waters of South Vietnam. Weapons and people were often hidden by civilians in sampans (a common type of Vietnamese boat), and the job of the US sailors was to halt and inspect all suspicious craft. Brown-water boats patrolled inland waterways, deltas, and coastal areas day and night and also enforced the nightly curfew on boat traffic.

A second mission was combat. A coordinated combat unit with Army personnel, the Army-Navy Riverine Assault Force, sought out and attacked enemy combatants on and along waterways and delta areas.

Among the many Brown Water Navy operations were Operation Game Warden (1965–1970), which was an interdiction effort focused on the inland waterways of South Vietnam; Operation Market Time, which dealt with interdiction on the coast and included Blue Water Navy ships; and Operation SEALORDS (Southeast Asia Lake, Ocean, River, and Delta Strategy) in the Mekong Delta.

The living conditions of brown-water sailors differed from those of the blue water sailors. For example, brown-water sailors typically lived onshore in temporary barracks or tents and sometimes on their boats if no safe onshore accommodations were available.

Although accurate information on the number of naval personnel considered to be in the Brown Water Navy is not available, the Commander US Naval Forces Vietnam Monthly Historical Summary for October 1969 indicates that on a typical day in March 1969 there were 160 river assault craft in operation, including Vietnamese Marine Corps craft (available at: http://www.history.navy.mil/ar/docs/comnavforv/1969/October1969.pdf). Given the complement of men aboard each vessel type, that could mean that more than 1,000 sailors were engaged in these operations, although this would not constitute the entire Brown Water Navy.

The Coast Guard in the Vietnam War

Over 8,000 Americans served in Vietnam as part of the Coast Guard. The Coast Guard operated under the authority of the Navy and served in five major categories of operations: preventing enemy and enemy-supply movement, port security, aids to navigation, ensuring the safe and efficient transport of supplies by merchant ships, and search and rescue. Some Coast Guard personnel served on small ships and boats that functioned as part of the Brown Water Navy; others served aboard larger ships, such as the high-endurance cutters, which had crews of around 100–150 men and were part of the Blue Water Navy fleet (Scotti, 2000). In the present report, the committee does not distinguish between Coast Guard and Navy sailors; the committee assumed that Coast Guard sailors would have the same exposure potentials as Blue Water Navy or Brown Water Navy sailors, depending on the types of activities they undertook and the types of ships or boats on which they served.

The Merchant Marine in the Vietnam War

During the Vietnam War, as in other wars, the US Merchant Marine functioned as an auxiliary of the Navy and transported supplies for the armed forces. Ships in the Merchant Marine are civilian owned and staffed by civilians, but Navy personnel were sometimes stationed aboard these ships. Merchant Marine vessels included both large oceangoing ships that took supplies across the Pacific from the United States or from Navy bases elsewhere in Asia, and smaller vessels that transported supplies upriver within Vietnam (American Merchant Marine at War, http://www.usmm.org/vietnam.html). Many materials, including herbicides, were shipped from the United States to Vietnam on civilian-manned Merchant Marine ships, not via Navy vessels. With the exception of some merchant seamen who served during World War II, members of the Merchant Marine are not recognized as military veterans and thus are not eligible for VA benefits (http://www.usmm.org/vietnam.html).

Land-Based Naval Operations in Vietnam

In South Vietnam, the Navy was active throughout the war in advising and training the South Vietnamese Navy. Navy personnel were also involved in humanitarian and morale-building campaigns. For example, hospital ships provided health care for the civilian South Vietnamese population both aboard ships and through outreach on land. The Seabees, the construction force of the Navy, lived ashore and constructed harbor facilities and engaged in other building projects. In general, these sailors experienced living conditions similar to those of noncombat personnel in the other services that were stationed in Vietnam on similar missions.

THE DEBATE OVER BLUE WATER NAVY EXPOSURE TO AGENT ORANGE

A variety of tactical herbicides were used by the American military in Vietnam during 1962–1971 to defoliate forests and destroy crops. Some of them, including the mixture known as Agent Orange, contained the highly toxic TCDD. The extent of herbicide spraying varied across the country, with some areas receiving far more extensive spraying than others. For example, during the Vietnam War the American military divided South Vietnam into four geographic zones (see Figure 2-1) and III Corps Area, which included the area around Saigon, was sprayed with more than twice as much herbicide as the other zones (IOM, 1994). (See Chapter 3 for more information on the herbicides, including the volumes sprayed in Vietnam.)

Agent Orange Legislation

By the middle 1950s, there was evidence from industrial exposures and accidents that the TCDD found in Agent Orange posed health risks for humans. During the Vietnam War, American scientists voiced concerns about possible health risks for American troops and the Vietnamese population, and the US government commissioned a series of studies on the issue in the mid- to late 1960s (Butler, 2005). On the basis of those studies, the United States in October 1969 began limiting its use of herbicides in Vietnam; spraying ceased entirely in 1971 (IOM, 1994).

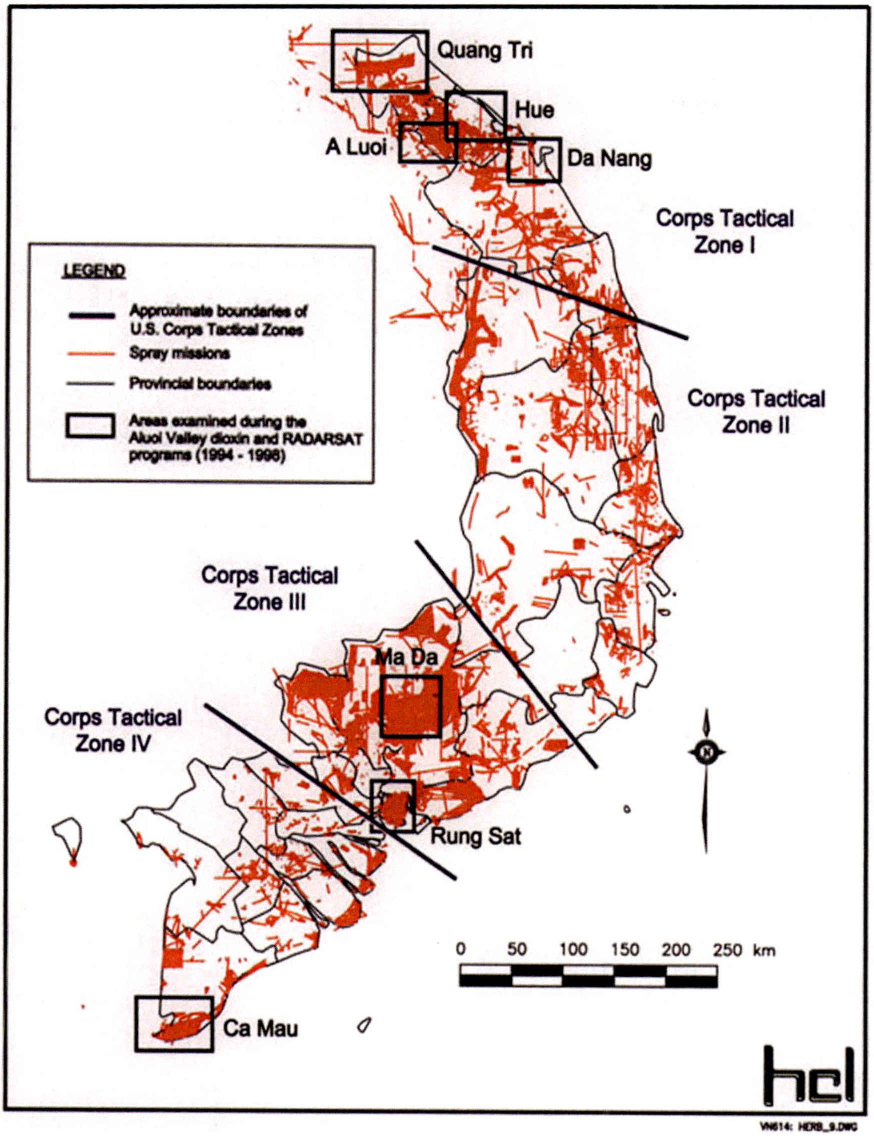

FIGURE 2-1 Aerial herbicide spraying missions in southern Vietnam, 1965–1971.
SOURCE: Reproduced with permission from Hatfield Consulting, http://www.cc.gatech.edu/~tpilsch/AirOps/Images/RanchHand/Map-spray_msns-RVN-65-71.jpg (accessed February 22, 2011).

Additional concerns about the health risks posed to Vietnam veterans arose after the war. In the late 1970s, a Chicago benefits counselor in the Veterans' Administration (now the Department of Veterans Affairs) began to suspect that Agent Orange was causing health problems in Vietnam veterans, and her testimony in the 1977 televised documentary *Agent Orange: The Deadly Fog* increased the general public's and veterans' awareness of the issue. In 1979, a class-action lawsuit was filed by veterans against several large chemical companies that had manufactured the herbicides used during the war. The case was settled out of court in 1984, and a settlement fund was established (Schuck, 1986).

Beginning in 1979, Congress enacted several laws to examine links between exposure to herbicides in Vietnam and possible long-term health effects. In 1984, Congress first required the VA to establish guidelines and standards for evaluating the scientific studies and to issue regulations for adjudicating claims for VA benefits based on herbicide exposure. In 1991, Public Law (PL) 102-4, the Agent Orange Act, was passed. It required VA to ask the IOM to conduct periodic reviews of the available scientific and medical evidence of health effects that followed exposure to the herbicides used in Vietnam, including Agent Orange and its contaminant TCDD. The law also stipulated that the IOM studies be conducted every 2 years for 10 years after publication of the initial report, which occurred in 1994. The Veteran Education and Benefits Expansion Act of 2001 (PL 107-103) extended the timeframe of the studies through 2014. Based on the eight biennial *Veterans and Agent Orange* (*VAO*) reports published to date that assessed the peer-reviewed literature on the health effects of exposure to herbicides, particularly Agent Orange and TCDD, the VA has identified 14 health conditions associated with Agent Orange exposure. For a discussion of those health effects, see Chapter 6 of the present report and the *VAO* report series.

The Blue Water Navy's Exposure to Tactical Herbicides During the Vietnam War

As with any war, it is difficult or impossible for those serving in the conflicts to identify the many chemical agents to which they might have been exposed intentionally or unintentionally during active duty. Because of the impossibility that most Vietnam veterans could prove that they had been exposed to Agent Orange or other herbicides in Vietnam during the war, the 1991 act created a presumption of service connection;

that is, exposure to herbicides in Vietnam was presumed for any Vietnam veteran who became ill with a disease found to be associated with TCDD exposure. That presumption—a mechanism of disability compensation that the VA has used in other contexts—allows veterans to receive disability compensation and treatment for a medical condition without having to provide proof that the condition was "incurred in or aggravated by" their military service (38 USC 1116(a)(2)).

As the VA began to process applications for presumptive service connections for herbicide-related disabilities, it was forced to decide whether service in the waters off the coast of Vietnam satisfied the requirements of the statute for service in Vietnam. The statutory language defines eligibility as extending to veterans "who, during active military, naval, or air service, served in the Republic of Vietnam during the period beginning on January 9, 1962, and ending on May 7, 1975" (USC 1116 (a)(1)). The decision of whether blue water service constituted service in the Republic of Vietnam was not consistent for a number of years. One commonly used standard for service "in the Republic of Vietnam" was possession of a Vietnam Service Medal, which was given to members of the Blue Water Navy who served in or near Vietnamese waters as part of the war effort. In 1997, the VA held that "service on a deep-water naval vessel in waters off the shore of the Republic of Vietnam does not constitute 'service in the Republic of Vietnam' for purposes of 38 U.S.C. § 101(29)(A) (VA, 1997)." As a result of that precedent opinion, at least some Blue Water Navy veterans who received Vietnam Service Medals were denied claims.

Haas v. Peake

Attention to whether Blue Water Navy Vietnam veterans were or should be eligible for a presumptive service connection to herbicide exposure increased as a result of a challenge to the VA precedent opinion in the court case *Haas v. Peake*. In 2001, Blue Water Navy Vietnam veteran Jonathan Haas first sought a presumptive service connection from his VA regional office for type II diabetes. Haas had served on the ammunition ship *USS Mount Katmai* off the coast of Vietnam during August 1967–April 1969. He had never gone ashore, and his ship had never gone into port in Vietnam, but he claimed that the *Mount Katmai* had sailed as close as 100 ft from the Vietnamese coast and had been "engulfed by an Agent Orange cloud" and thus argued that he had been exposed (*Haas v. Peake*. 2008. Jonathan L. Haas, Claimant-Appellee v.

James B. Peake, Secretary of Veterans Affairs, Respondent-Appellant. 2007-7037. US Court of Appeals for the Federal Circuit.). When his claim was denied, he appealed the regional office decision to the Board of Veterans' Appeals, where it was again denied in 2004.

In denying his claim, the board in 2004 cited the regulatory language in the *Code of Federal Regulations* (*CFR*), which stated that "service in the Republic of Vietnam includes service in the waters offshore and service in other locations if the conditions of service involved duty or visitation in the Republic of Vietnam" (CFR Title 38, 3.307(a)4(iii)), and Haas had not served on the ground or on the inland waters. The court also stated in its decision that his claim was rejected because it was "unsupported by any evidence demonstrating that this ship was located in waters sprayed by herbicides."

Haas again appealed, and this time the VA decision was reversed by the US Court of Appeals for Veterans Claims (*Haas v. Nicholson*. 2006. Jonathan L. Haas, Appellant v. R. James Nicholson, Secretary of Veterans Affairs, Appellee. No. 04-0491. United States Court of Appeals for Veterans Claims.). That court, known as the Veterans Court, found the VA's interpretation of the regulatory language defining service in Vietnam as requiring service on inland waters or on Vietnamese soil to be unduly restrictive. The court also cited the VA's history of granting presumptive service connections for members of the Blue Water Navy who had received Vietnam Service Medals and commented on the issue of whether exposure was possible:

> Given the spraying of Agent Orange along the coastline and the wind borne effects of such spraying, it appears that these veterans serving on vessels in close proximity to land would have the same risk of exposure to the herbicide Agent Orange as veterans serving on adjacent land, or an even greater risk than that borne by those veterans who may have visited and set foot on the land of the Republic of Vietnam only briefly (*Haas v. Nicholson*. 2006. Jonathan L. Haas, Appellant v. R. James Nicholson, Secretary of Veterans Affairs, Appellee. No. 04-0491. United States Court of Appeals for Veterans Claims.).

The VA appealed the decision and in 2008, the Veterans Court decision was reversed, and the VA's original decision to deny a presumption of service connection to Blue Water Navy veterans was upheld by the US Court of Appeals for the Federal Circuit (*Haas v. Peake*. 2008. Jonathan L. Haas, Claimant-Appellee v. James B. Peake,

Secretary of Veterans Affairs, Respondent-Appellant. 2007-7037. US Court of Appeals for the Federal Circuit.). The US Court of Appeals found the VA's interpretation of service in Vietnam to require visitation to land or travel on inland waterways to be permissible. The court did not find the decision to exclude Blue Water veterans to be arbitrary and concluded that because the VA general counsel's interpretation of the regulatory language was "neither plainly erroneous nor inconsistent with the language of the regulation," it deserved judicial deference by the appeals court (*Haas v. Peake.* May 8, 2008. Decision Assessment Document. No. 2007-7307. 2008. United States Court of Appeals for the Federal Court.).

During the appeal process for the Haas case, there was a court-ordered stay on processing Blue Water veterans' claims, many of which had been made after the 2006 Veterans Court decision. After the final decision in 2008 (the Supreme Court declined to hear the case), the VA began processing the backlog of 17,000 claims, most of which were from Blue Water Navy Vietnam veterans. Although these veterans were not eligible for an automatic presumption, each case needed to be reviewed to determine whether a nonpresumptive service connection was justified or the veteran in question actually qualified for the presumption because his boat docked or entered Vietnamese inland waters while he was aboard.

Royal Australian Navy

The original Haas claim cited direct spraying and aerial drift of herbicides as possible routes of exposure for Blue Water Navy personnel off the coast of Vietnam. In the 2008 court proceedings, a new route of possible exposure was introduced: the ingestion of TCDD through contaminated potable water on Blue Water Navy ships. This claim was based on the results of a study commissioned by the Australian Department of Veterans Affairs in 2002 that suggested that the water-distillation process used aboard Australian Navy ships could result in increased concentrations of TCDD in the potable water made on the ship (Muller et al., 2002). That study had been prompted by the finding that mortality in Royal Australian Navy (RAN) veterans was higher than that in Australian veterans who served on the ground in Vietnam during the war (see Chapter 6 for a more detailed discussion of this epidemiologic study). On the basis of the epidemiologic results and the 2002 Australian distillation study, the Australian Department of Veterans Affairs decided to provide disability compensation to its Vietnam naval veterans for medical conditions related to herbicide exposure.

The IOM committee that prepared the most recent *VAO* report (IOM, 2009) examined the validity of those findings and how they might relate to the potential for the US Navy water-distillation systems to concentrate TCDD and found them to be scientifically reasonable. Inasmuch as US Navy ships used the same distillation systems as the RAN, the committee concluded

> No measurements of TCDD concentrations in seawater were collected during the Vietnam conflict, so it is not possible to ascertain the extent to which drinking water on US vessels may have been contaminated through distillation processes. However, it seems likely that vessels with such distillation processes that traveled near land or even at some distance from river deltas would periodically collect water that contained dioxin. Thus, a presumption of exposure of military personnel serving on those vessels is not unreasonable. (IOM, 2009)

The presence of TCDD in shipboard potable water requires the assumption that TCDD was present in the marine water used to distill the potable water. The Australian study cited accounts from Australian sailors who served on RAN ships, that the ships frequently drew marine water in or near the mouths of estuaries and river deltas to make potable water and used marine water from the open ocean to make distilled water to run the boilers; the boilers required far more distilled water than did the ships' crews. Subsequent information received from the Australian Department of Veterans Affairs indicated that although RAN standard operating procedures required that, except in emergency circumstances, potable water was to be made only when 10 or more miles from populated shores, these procedures were not always followed and the reasons for doing so were not clear (Eileen Wilson, Australian Department of Veterans Affairs, personal communication, October 10, 2010). Four RAN ships provided support to US Navy ships on gunlines that could be located as close as 2.8 miles (4,572 meters) from the coast; the ships spent about one month on the gunline (Wilson et al., 2005a).

Current Status of Blue Water Navy Veterans' Claims

VA continues to deny Blue Water Navy Vietnam veterans presumptions of service connections for herbicide-related conditions unless

> for those Veterans who served aboard ships that docked and the Veteran went ashore, or served aboard ships that did not dock but the Veteran went ashore, their service involved "visitation" in Vietnam. In cases involving docking, the evidence must show that the Veteran was aboard at the time of docking and the Veteran must provide a statement of personally going ashore. In cases where shore docking did not occur, the evidence must show that the ship operated in Vietnam's close coastal waters for extended periods, that members of the crew went ashore, or that smaller vessels from the ship went ashore regularly with supplies or personnel. In these cases, the Veteran must also provide a statement of personally going ashore. (VA, 1997)

The VA continues to develop a list of Blue Water Navy ships documented to have entered inland waters and the dates on which they did so. A ship that was in a deep-water harbor, for example, such as Da Nang, would not count as being in "brown water" (VA, 2008).

The largest Blue Water Navy ships, the aircraft carriers, rarely entered inland waters or came close enough to shore to dock due to their large size and vulnerability to enemy attack. Cruisers also were too large to enter inland waterways, although a few did enter some sections of rivers such as the Saigon and the Cua Viet. Smaller ship classes such as destroyers, destroyer escorts, minesweepers, survey ships, salvage ships, cargo and transport ships were capable of safely navigating some inland waterways and did so on occasion as part of their military missions. As of January 2011, over 140 individual ships and 51 classes of Navy vessels that served in the Seventh Fleet during the Vietnam era have been categorized as having served primarily or exclusively in inland waterways, temporarily in inland waterways, or in coastal waterways of Vietnam with evidence that crew members went ashore or that smaller ships regularly went ashore with supplies or personnel (James Sampsel, VA, personal communication, January 12, 2011).

Blue Water Vietnam veterans can still file claims for service-related disabilities, but their claims have to be reviewed case by case and exposure to herbicides has to be demonstrated. Blue Water Navy veterans are eligible for compensation under a separate regulation for non-Hodgkin's lymphoma (NHL). Under 38 CFR 3.313, "service in Vietnam" includes service in waters offshore for the purposes of NHL compensation, because there is no claim of a link to herbicide exposure.

Underlying the controversy of Blue Water Navy Vietnam veterans' claims to a presumption of herbicide exposure are the legal mandates to compensate veterans for their current health problems. Vietnam veterans who served on the ground and on the inland waterways of Vietnam are eligible for compensation for their health problems regardless of the time they spent in Vietnam and the potential for their exposure to the tactical herbicides, such as Agent Orange, that were widely used during the war.

REFERENCES

Appy, C. G. 1993. *Working-class war: American combat soldiers & Vietnam.* Chapel Hill, NC: University of North Carolina Press.

Butler, D. A. 2005. Connections: The early history of scientific and medical research on "Agent Orange." *Journal of Law and Policy* 13:527-552.

IOM (Institute of Medicine). 1994. *Veterans and Agent Orange: Health effects of herbicides used in Vietnam.* Washington, DC: National Academy Press.

IOM. 2009. *Veterans and Agent Orange: Update 2008.* Washington, DC: The National Academies Press.

Marolda, E. J. 1994. *By sea, air, and land: An illustrated history of the U.S. Navy and the war in Southeast Asia.* Washington, DC: Naval Historical Center.

Muller, J. F., C. Gaus, K. Bundred, V. Alberts, M. R. Moore, and K. Horsley. 2002. *Examination of the potential exposure of Royal Australian Navy (RAN) personnel to polychlorinated dibenzo TCDDs and polychlorinated dibenzofurans via drinking water. A report to: The Department of Veteran Affairs, Australia.* Brisbane, Australia: National Research Centre for Environmental Toxicology.

Schuck, P. H. 1986. *Agent Orange on trial: Mass toxic disasters in the courts.* Cambridge, MA: Belknap Press of Harvard University Press.

Scotti, P. C. 2000. *Coast Guard action in Vietnam: Stories of those who served.* Central Point, OR: Hellgate Press.

Turley, W. S. 2009. *The second Indochina war: A concise political and military history,* 2nd ed. Lanham, MD: Rowman & Littlefield Publishers.

VA (Department of Veterans Affairs). 1997. *Service in the Republic of Vietnam for purposes of definition of Vietnam Era—38 U.S.C. § 101(29)(A). Memorandum from VA General Counsel to Director of Compensation and Pension Service.* VAOPGCPREC 27-97. July 23, 1997.

VA. 2008. Further definition of Vietnam "Blue Water" versus "Brown Water" service for the purpose of determining Agent Orange exposure. *Compensation & Pension Service Bulletin* p. 2-3. December.

3

SELECTED CHEMICALS USED DURING THE VIETNAM WAR

This chapter discusses three groups of chemicals used by the US military in Vietnam. First and in greatest depth, the committee reviews the use of tactical herbicides, such as Agent Orange, which is the focus of this report. Second, some other chemicals used abundantly by the US military during the war—including such nontactical pesticides as malathion, and jet and diesel fuels—are described. Finally, Blue Water Navy and Brown Water Navy personnel were exposed to many chemicals that were needed to operate and maintain their ships. Exposure opportunity varied greatly with a sailor's occupation, the class of ship, and the activity that required the use of the chemical(s). Many of the chemicals used aboard are known to be toxic and can result in both short-term and long-term adverse health effects. Because naval personnel are known to have been exposed to at least some of these chemicals during their tours of duty in Vietnam, the committee found it important to identify and describe a few of the chemicals, their uses, and their long-term health effects.

HERBICIDE USE IN VIETNAM

During the Vietnam War (1962–1975), both the US and the Republic of Vietnam militaries used several herbicides for tactical purposes, specifically to defoliate areas to reduce cover for enemy forces, to improve visibility on the perimeters of military installations, and for a short time to kill enemy crops. Both the US Air Force and the US Army Chemical Corps purchased herbicides and used them in Vietnam. Different tactical herbicides were used at different times during the war (Young, 2009). By far the most widely used herbicide was Agent Orange, followed by Agent White; other tactical herbicides that were used in Vietnam during the war include Agent Blue, Agent Purple, Agent Pink, and Agent Green. The names of the herbicides were derived from the color-coded bands around the 55-gal (208-L) drums used to ship and store them (Young, 2009). The military use of herbicides has been discussed in several other Institute of Medicine (IOM) reports (IOM, 1994, 2003, 2008) and two books (Buckingham, 1983; Young, 2009), and will not be described in detail here.

The tactical herbicides used in Vietnam were intended to kill a broad spectrum of plants. Agent Orange and Agent White were used against broadleaf plants and woody shrubs and trees, including mangroves. Agent Blue was effective against grasses and grains, such as rice (Young, 2009).

Herbicide Composition

2,4,5-Trichlorophenoxyacetic acid (2,4,5-T) was the main active ingredient of Agent Orange and the herbicides used earlier in the Vietnam War. As a result of the synthesis of 2,4,5-T, it was contaminated with 2,3,7,8-tetrachlorodibenzo-p-dioxin (2,3,7,8-TCDD, also referred to as TCDD). Production of 2,4,5-T ceased in 1979 when the US Environmental Protection Agency (EPA) canceled all registrations for its use (EPA, 1979). The EPA based that decision on its toxicity resulting from its unavoidable TCDD contamination. Of the herbicides used in Vietnam, only those containing 2,4,5-T were contaminated with TCDD. 2,4-dichlorophenoxyacetic acid (2,4-D)—a second active ingredient of Agent Orange, Agent White, and Agent Purple—was and continues to be a widely used herbicide around the world. Its human health and environmental risks were assessed by the EPA in 2005 to support its reregistration. It is permitted for agricultural and residential herbicide use (EPA, 2005).

The magnitude of TCDD contamination in the herbicides used in Vietnam is the subject of controversy. Part of the issue is that the herbicides were not tested for TCDD content when manufactured or used. Assessment of TCDD content is based on the analysis of the herbicide stockpiles that were stored at Johnston Island in the Pacific and the Naval Construction Battalion Center in Gulfport, Mississippi, before their destruction by at-sea incineration in 1977. The TCDD content was known to vary by herbicide and by production run. Some manufacturers were able to reduce the TCDD concentrations in their 2,4,5-T during the 1960s, particularly after 1967 when one manufacturer installed an activated carbon filter (Piacitelli et al., 2000); other manufacturers also reduced the TCDD contamination of their 2,4,5-T by about 1968 (Young, 2009). Stellman et al. (2003) reports that TCDD concentrations in Agent Orange ranged from 6.2 to 14.3 ppm (average, 13.25 ppm), but other ranges have been estimated on the basis of other herbicide samples, for example, less than 0.05 to 17.0 ppm (NAS, 1974), and the levels reported by Young (2009) in Table 3-1. Agent Purple was likely to have been even more highly contaminated with TCDD than Agent Orange (Stellman et al., 2003), containing up to 45 ppm TCDD. It is also likely that the herbicides used earlier in the war, such as Agent Pink, were more highly contaminated with TCDD. Stellman et al. (2003) calculated that 221 kg of TCDD was sprayed in Vietnam by US forces, and this does not include herbicides used by the Vietnamese forces or herbicides sprayed other than by C-123 aircraft. Young (2009) reported that 105–119 kg of TCDD were sprayed by US forces, based on his lower estimates of TCDD contamination of Agent Orange.

Agent Orange, the most widely used herbicide in Vietnam, was soluble in diesel fuel and organic solvents but not soluble in water. Agent White, in contrast, was soluble in water but not soluble in diesel fuel or organic solvents. Agent Blue was a powder that was mixed with water before application; the formulation contained organic pentavalent arsenic (Young, 2009). According to Young (2009), all the tactical herbicides used in Vietnam were applied in concentrated form and not diluted.

Intentional Release of Herbicides in Vietnam

It has been estimated that over 74 million liters of tactical herbicides were used in Vietnam during 1961–1971, of which Agent Orange made up almost 60% (43 million liters) (see Table 3-1). The amount of Agent Orange sprayed varied by military region: I Corps south of the demilitarized zone–8.52 million liters; II Corps–9.54 million liters; III Corps near Saigon–20.1 million liters, and IV Corps in the Mekong Delta region–4.66 million liters (IOM, 1994). The herbicides were purchased from several US chemical manufacturers and transported via commercial Merchant Marine ships from the United States to military installations in Vietnam. Blue Water Navy and Coast Guard vessels were not used to transport herbicides from the United States to the Republic of Vietnam (Baldini, 2009). The US Air Force's Operation Ranch Hand was the military code name for the US Air Force's spraying of herbicides in Vietnam from 1962 to 1971, when the operation was discontinued.

TABLE 3-1 Major Herbicides Used in Operation Ranch Hand, 1962–1971

Code Name	Formulation	Amount Sprayed in Vietnam, liters	Period of Use	TCDD Concentration
Green	2,4,5-T	75,920	1962–1964	65.6 ppm
Pink	2,4,5-T	273,520	1962–1964	65.6 ppm
Purple	2,4-D, 2,4,5-T	2,594,800	1962–1964	Up to 45 ppm
Blue	Cacodylic acid (4.7%), sodium cacodylate (26.4%)	6,100,640	1962–1971	None
Orange I, Orange II	2,4-D (50%), 2,4,5-T (50%)	43,332,640	1965–1970	0.05–50 ppm (average, 1.98–2.99 ppm)
White	2,4-D (39.6%), picloram (10.2%)	21,798,400	1965–1971	None

SOURCE: Young (2009).

Operation Ranch Hand was responsible for the spraying of more than 95% of all herbicides used in Vietnam; spraying was done from modified C-123 aircraft (Stellman et al., 2003; Young, 2009). Defoliation occurred along waterways, roads, railroads, and other transportation routes to lower the risk of ambush. Extensive spraying was also conducted in the Mekong River delta area around the coastal mangrove swamps, also with the goal of reducing protective cover for the enemy. Operation Ranch Hand peaked in 1967, when 1.7 million acres of Vietnam and Laos were sprayed, 85% for defoliation and 15% for crop destruction.

A small proportion of the herbicides was applied by other means, such as backpacks, spray trucks, helicopters, and boats. The US Army Chemical Corps ground personnel sprayed herbicides from trucks or backpacks around base perimeters; other Army personnel sprayed herbicides from helicopters (Darrow, 1969) and directly from drums along waterways (Marolda, 1994). Members of the Army Chemical Corps reported spraying herbicides, handling spray equipment, being present when others were spraying, getting herbicides on their skin or clothing, and passing through defoliated areas (Kang et al., 2001). The Air Force maintained a record of spraying missions from August 1965 to December 1971 in the Herbicide Reporting System (HERBS) files. From 1968 to 1971, the HERBS files also contained information on the US Army helicopter spraying missions. The US Navy sprayed herbicides along river banks (Darrow, 1969), but the committee was unable to locate any specific information on Navy herbicide spraying on inland waterways in Vietnam.

Land-Based Application

The Ranch Hand C-123 aircraft had herbicide spray apparatus with nozzles that produced droplets measuring 320–350 μm with rapid settling velocity (Young et al., 2004b). A full tank sprayed a swath 80 m wide and 14 km long in 3.5–4 min. The average deposit was 2.9 mL/m^2 (3 gal/acre). Virtually all droplets, even those smaller than 100 μm, were estimated to intercept the target area within 3 min, and 87% of the Agent Orange would hit vegetation within 1 min; the remaining 13% of the herbicide would not contact vegetation within the designated swath and thus would drift as droplets or volatilize into the gas phase of air (Young, 2009).

The Ranch Hand aircraft sprayed from 50 m above the ground. Environmental conditions for a mission included inversion or neutral atmospheric conditions, that is, wind less than 10 knots (0.005 km/s) at ground level with flight paths oriented into the wind as much as possible, temperature below 29°C (missions were typically flown early in the morning), no rain or predicted rain, and good visibility. Multiple aircraft, up to eight, were used for some spray missions, although 70% of the missions involved three or fewer aircraft (Stellman et al., 2003; Young, 2009). The HERBS file for Operation Ranch Hand contains the most comprehensive data on the herbicide missions flown in Vietnam, including flight date, flight path, turning points and markers for activation and deactivation of spray apparatus, herbicide used, and aircraft type. After review and corrections, 9,141 missions are recorded in the HERBS file, including 1,081 ground missions and 2,108 helicopter missions (Jeanne Stellman, Columbia University, personal communications, October 21 and October 28, 2010). These missions included fighter support aircraft for protection against enemy fire (Young, 2009).

Land-based application via helicopters, trucks, and backpacks was conducted at lower speeds and lower altitudes (for helicopters) for base perimeter defoliation, roadside spraying, and some crop destruction. The Army Chemical Corps was responsible for these applications, which accounted for about 3–4% of the herbicide used in Vietnam. The buffalo turbine mounted on trucks could disperse herbicide at 280 m^3/min and cover a swath 75 m wide. Backpack units held 11 L of herbicide.

As noted by both Stellman et al. (2003 and presentation to committee) and Young (2009), the flight paths of the C-123s often included flying over rivers, streams, and delta areas with direct application of Agent Orange or other herbicides to the water surface. An additional method of herbicide application was direct spraying by the Brown Water Navy on riverbanks. Although the committee heard several reports of such spraying and there is a video of it on the Internet (http://www.youtube.com/watch?v=wUZA0GAMmfI), the committee was unable to locate much documentation of the practice (Darrow, 1969) or to determine how much Agent Orange or other herbicides were applied.

Dumping of Herbicides in Coastal Waters

On the basis of the revised HERBS files, Stellman et al. (2003) reported that 42 missions, totaling about 120,000 L of herbicide, are known to have resulted in emergency herbicide dumps. Stellman et al. noted that "aborted missions may not represent the significant source of exposure." Only a few of the 42 missions that dumped herbicides appear to have been near the coast of South Vietnam (Jeanne Stellman, Columbia University, personal communication, November 1, 2010). The Army also verified that some herbicide was jettisoned over water near the Vietnamese coast (Department of the Army, 1981). The committee did not attempt to identify where each aborted or jettisoned missions occurred; this information may be contained in an uncorrected version of the HERBS file, known as the Map Book.

OTHER CHEMICAL-EXPOSURE OPPORTUNITIES

In addition to tactical herbicides, C-123s operating over Vietnam sprayed other pesticides. One of the banes of tropical warfare is malaria. In an effort to control the incidence of malaria in US ground troops in Vietnam, the military initiated Operation Flyswatter (Cecil and Young, 2008). That program, which began in 1967, used modified Ranch Hand C-123 aircraft, also known as Bug Birds, to spray malathion. Unlike the C-123s used for herbicide spraying, the Bug Birds flew alone without escort aircraft and were not camouflaged. Malathion was stored at Bien Hoa Air Base, Cam Ranh Bay Air Base, and Da Nang Air Base. Initially, the pesticide was sprayed over nine major US bases and adjacent sites every 11–14 days. Spraying typically was conducted 1.5 hr after dawn and 1.5 hr before sunset. Malathion in a 57% concentrate (later 95%) was applied at 0.59 L/hectare. Environmental conditions were similar to those used for herbicide spraying—maximum winds of 10 knots (0.005 km/s), maximum temperature of 30°C, and no rainfall during or for 1 hr after spraying. Aircraft flew at 45 m above the ground at an air speed of 130 knots to cover about 6,000 hectares on one sortie (Cecil and Young, 2008). In all, Operation Flyswatter sprayed more that 1.76 million liters of malathion over about 6 million hectares in South Vietnam (Young et al., 2004a). Cecil and Young (2008) report that that was about half the total insecticides used by all forces during the war. Short-term exposure to high concentrations of malathion has been shown to produce disturbances to various organ systems including the following: gastrointestinal system (vomiting, cramps, diarrhea); respiratory system (difficulty breathing, chest tightness); and central nervous system (watery eyes, blurred vision, salivation, sweating, headaches, dizziness, loss of consciousness, and death) (ATSDR, 2003).

US military personnel in Vietnam also had substantial opportunity for exposure to diesel fuel. Diesel fuel was used not only for operating equipment and vehicles. JP-8 and JP-4, for instance, are types of diesel fuel used for aircraft such as jets and Huey helicopters. The committee heard reports that many of Navy personnel aboard aircraft carriers were frequently sprayed with jet fuel. Naval tankers delivered large amounts of diesel fuel to ground forces. Breathing fuel oils such as diesel fuel may result in short-term adverse effects, such as eye irritation, nausea, and headache; long-term exposure to diesel fuel fumes may result in kidney damage and loss of the blood's ability to clot (ATSDR, 1995).

CHEMICALS USED ABOARD US NAVY SHIPS

Blue Water Navy and Brown Water Navy personnel were exposed to many chemicals during their shipboard deployments. Exposure may have occurred by ingestion, inhalation, or dermal contact.

Some common chemicals found aboard surface vessels and their potential associated adverse health effects are presented in Table 3-2. The table is not meant to be comprehensive but rather represents some of the chemicals to which naval personnel might have been exposed while serving on ships in the Blue Water Navy during the Vietnam War. In

TABLE 3-2 Examples of Adverse Health Effects Associated with Chemical Exposure

Chemical	Use Category	Adverse Health Effect[a]
Polychlorinated biphenyls[b]	Insulation	Cancer
Trichloroethylene[c]	Degreaser	Cancer
Mercury[d]	Explosives, disinfectants, batteries	Peripheral neuropathy
Benzene[e]	Component of jet and other fuels, combustion product, cigarette smoke	Leukemia
Phosgene[c]	Welding	Chronic obstructive pulmonary disease
Asbestos[b]	Insulation, cement pipe, sealants, plasters	Cancer, pulmonary disease, asbestosis
Hydraulic fluids[c]	Machinery lubricants	Nervous system effects
Lead[b]	Paint, cable and wire, plastics, pastes, caulks	Neuropathy
Hydrazine[f]	Electroplating, soldering, boiler water	Neurotoxicity

[a]Long-term adverse health effects from Haz-Map Database, National Library of Medicine.
[b]Navy Occupational Safety and Health Program Manual for Forces Afloat. Volume I. SOH and Major Hazard-Specific Programs (Department of the Navy, 2002).
[c]Trichloroethylene factsheet. Available at: http://www.nmcphc.med.navy.mil/downloads/ep/factsheets/tce.pdf (accessed January 19, 2011).
[d]Navy Occupational Safety and Health Program Manual for Forces Afloat. Volume II. Surface Ship Safety Standards (Department of the Navy, 2007).
[e]Benzene factsheet: Available at: http://www.nmcphc.med.navy.mil/downloads/ep/factsheets/benzene.pdf (accessed January 19, 2011).
[f]Navy MIL-H-24776: Hydrazine Test Kit, Naval Shipboard. 1992. Available at: http://engineers.ihs.com/document/abstract/NCSWDAAAAAAAAAA (accessed January 19, 2011).

determining long-term adverse health effects of chemicals like those shown in Table 3-2, it is generally presumed that a person was exposed to a single chemical. However, in practice, personnel aboard naval vessels were exposed to a complex mixture of environmental contaminants. Those exposures could occur concurrently or sequentially. The importance of understanding the exposures is twofold. First, the long-term adverse health effects of some of the chemicals are similar to those associated with exposure to dioxins, such as some cancers (for example, TCDD and benzene with leukemia) and peripheral neuropathy (for example, TCDD and mercury). A cancer induced by a shipboard chemical exposure cannot be differentiated from a similar cancer produced by TCDD, particularly given the multitude of chemical exposures that most people experience and the long latent period of most cancers. Second, chemicals in a mixture may antagonize or synergize each other's effects. For example, exposure to one chemical may make a person more susceptible or more resistant to the effect of a second chemical. If exposure to two chemicals is concurrent, it may result in an additive, synergistic, or antagonistic effect. It is noteworthy that sailors on naval vessels were exposed not only to a mixture of chemicals as a result of their occupations and the ventilation systems but to chemicals in cigarette smoke, which render smokers (as well as nonsmokers exposed to secondhand smoke) more susceptible to other chemicals (Hoffmann and Hoffmann, 1997; Goud and Kaplan, 1999). The chemical composition of a mixture may change as components degrade or interact with each other, or as a result of different manufacturing conditions (for example, TCDD concentrations varied from batch to batch during production of Agent Orange). All those factors may affect the chemical mixtures to which sailors were exposed aboard naval vessels and thus affect their susceptibility to TCDD and other chemical exposures.

Several factors influence the potential for exposure to chemicals both onboard ships and shoreside. Among them are the class and mission of a ship, the ventilation system on the ship, and the use of multiple chemicals. Events such as shipboard transformer fires can also expose crewmembers to chemicals such as PCBs. Still et al. (2003) assessed PCB exposures on Navy surface ships and submarines, some dating to the Vietnam War. Although PCBs were not detected in any air samples taken on the surface ships, they were detected at 3,600 ppm in felt gasket material collected in the ventilation duct extraction system.

Many chemicals are used aboard ships in numerous occupational activities. In general, larger ships will have more chemicals onboard than smaller ships because there are more occupational activities on larger ships. For example, an aircraft carrier is essentially a floating industrial community, and the number of chemicals found onboard would be much higher than on a destroyer. An aircraft carrier would have chemicals onboard associated with the flying and maintenance of jet aircraft, whereas a destroyer or ammunition ship would not have such chemicals onboard. However, many of the chemicals would be comparable onboard all classes of ships. For example, a degreaser used by machinists onboard aircraft carriers could also be used by machinists onboard destroyers or frigates.

Navy enlisted classifications (NECs) for naval surface ships include a wide array of occupations, from aerographer and construction electrician to hull maintenance technician, machinist's mate, and yeoman. However, it is difficult to identify all the chemicals to which a person with a given NEC might be exposed during occupational activity; furthermore, there is the possibility that other naval personnel may inadvertently be exposed to some chemicals even if they are not working directly with them, mainly because of the ventilation system onboard Navy ships.

Navy shipboard living and working conditions differ considerably from those found shoreside. Shipboard environments are influenced by ventilation systems that run throughout the entire ship. The systems have the potential to spread airborne materials collected at one site to other sites throughout the ship if not properly designed and maintained. The potential spread of occupationally produced airborne materials could have a serious influence on the health of shipboard personnel. If the ventilation system is isolating individual work activities, personnel in the area would potentially be exposed only to the chemicals used in that area. However, if the ventilation system is not functioning properly, vapors and other airborne materials from other work areas could also be present; this can result in mixing of chemicals from different work areas with resultant exposures to complex mixtures by personnel onboard the ship.

Shoreside personnel conducting work similar to that found onboard ships may be using the same industrial chemicals but work under different environmental conditions. The activities often have different types of ventilation systems, both mechanical and natural. A shoreside welder may work in an area that has both local exhaust ventilation and natural ventilation, which is provided by open windows and doors. A shipboard welder typically does not have the luxury of an open window. If welding is conducted on deck, there is ample natural ventilation, but if the work is conducted below deck, natural ventilation is not available, so the shipboard welder is potentially exposed to a greater variety and higher concentrations of chemicals if not properly protected. Furthermore, there is considerable variation in environmental conditions for shoreside Navy personnel and, unlike shipboard naval personnel, they are less likely to spend both work time and leisure time in the same environment.

Naval ships and shore activities undergo numerous types of evaluations and inspections that establish actual or potential hazardous situations. Before the inception of specific Occupational Safety and Health Administration (OSHA) or EPA inspections, the naval medical department conducted comparable inspections; a ship the size of an aircraft carrier has a fully complemented medical department, including environmental-health personnel, who in earlier days provided comparable industrial-hygiene support. The Navy has conducted safety and occupational health programs for many years. Those programs gained special prominence after passage of the Occupational Safety and Health Act (OSHAct) in 1970. The primary thrust of the OSHAct was directed at private-sector employers; however, Section 19 of the OSHAct and several later presidential executive orders directed federal agencies to establish and maintain occupational safety and health programs. Requirements for such programs are contained in Title 29 of the Code of Federal Regulations, Part 1960 (29 CFR 1960). OPNAVINST 5100.19 series addresses the shipboard environment. Inspections would have been conducted by a ship's medical personnel, Navy hospital personnel, Navy Environmental Preventive Medicine Units or the equivalent, type commands, fleet commands, the Naval Safety Center (which was established in 1968), the Board of Inspection and Survey, or the systems commands (for example, NavSea and NavAir).

REFERENCES

ATSDR (Agency for Toxic Substances and Disease Registry). 1995. *Public health statement for fuel oils.* http://www.atsdr.cdc.gov/phs/phs.asp?id=514&tid=91 (accessed February 15, 2011).

ATSDR. 2003. *Public health statement for malathion.* http://www.atsdr.cdc.gov/phs/phs.asp?id=520&tid=92 (accessed February 15, 2011).

Baldini, D. 2009. *Memorandum for record: Joint Services Records Research Center statement on research findings regarding Navy and Coast Guard ships during the Vietnam era.* Alexandria, VA: Department of the Army, U.S. Army and Joint Services Records Research Center. May 1.

Brent, R. E., D. E. Rollins, D. P. Duffy, and M. C. Gregory. 1985. Standardized treatment of severe methanol poisoning with ethanol and hemodialysis. *Western Journal of Medicine* 142(3):337-340.

Buckingham, W. A. 1983. Operation Ranch Hand: Herbicides in Southeast Asia. *Air University Review*, July-August. 12 pgs. http://www.airpower.maxwell.af.mil/airchronicles/aureview/1983/jul-aug/buckingham.html (accessed October 18, 2010).

Cecil, P. F., and A. L. Young. 2008. Operation FLYSWATTER: A war within a war. *Environmental Science and Pollution Research* 15(1): 3-7.

Darrow, R. A. 1969. *Report of trip to Republic of Vietnam, 15 August-2 September 1969*. Department of the Army.

Department of the Army. 1981. Table, all MACV fixed wing aircraft herbicide incidents, 15 October 1981. Alexandria, VA: Department of the Army, Office of the Adjutant General.

Department of the Navy. 2002. *Navy Occupational Safety and Health Program manual for forces afloat. Volume I. SOH and Major Hazard-Specific Programs*. OPNAV Instruction 5100.19E. Washington, DC: Office of the Chief of Naval Operations.

Department of the Navy. 2007. *Navy Occupational Safety and Health Program manual for forces afloat. Volume II. Surface Ship Safety Standards*. OPNAV Instruction 5100.19E. Washington, DC: Office of the Chief of Naval Operations.

EPA (Environmental Protection Agency). 1979. *Decision and emergency order suspending registration for the forest, rights-of-way, and pasture uses of 2,4,5-trichlorophenoxyacetic acid (2,4,5-T)*. Washington, DC: Office of Pesticide Programs.

EPA. 2005. Reregistration eligibility decision for 2,4-D. Washington, DC: Office of Pesticide Programs.

Goud, S. N., and A. M. Kaplan. 1999. Inhibition of natural killer cell activity in mice treated with tobacco-specific carcinogen NNK. *Journal of Toxicology and Environmental Health* 56:131-144.

Hoffmann, D. , and I. Hoffmann. 1997. The changing cigarette 1950-1995. *Journal of Toxicology and Environmental Health* 50:307-364.

IOM (Institute of Medicine). 1994. *Veterans and Agent Orange: Health effects of herbicides used in Vietnam*. Washington, DC: National Academy Press.

IOM. 2003. *Characterizing exposure of veterans to Agent Orange and other herbicides used in Vietnam*. Washington, DC: The National Academies Press.

IOM. 2008. *The utility of proximity-based herbicide exposure assessment in epidemiologic studies of Vietnam veterans*. Washington, DC: The National Academies Press.

Kang, H. K., N. A. Dalager, L. L. Needham, D. G. Patterson, G. M. Matanoski, S. Kanchanaraksa, and P. S. J. Lees. 2001. US Army Chemical Corps Vietnam Veterans Health Study: Preliminary results. *Chemosphere* 43:943-949.

Marolda, E. J. 1994. *By sea, air, and land: An illustrated history of the U.S. Navy and the war in Southeast Asia*. Washington: Naval Historical Center.

NAS (National Academy of Sciences). 1974. *The effects of herbicides in South Vietnam*. Washington, DC: National Academy of Sciences.

Piacitelli, L., D. Marlow, M. Fingerhut, K. Steenland, and M. H. Sweeney. 2000. A retrospective job exposure matrix for estimating exposure to 2,3,7,8-tetrachloredibenzo-p-dioxin. *American Journal of Industrial Medicine* 38(1):28-39.

Somers, E. 1987. Modulation of response: Environmental factors. In *Methods for Assessing the Effects of Mixtures of Chemicals*, edited by V. B. Vouk, G. C. Butler, A. C. Upton, D. V. Parke and S. C. Asher. Chichester, UK: Scientific Committee on Problems of the Environment (SCOPE 30). http://globalecology.stanford.edu/ SCOPE/SCOPE_30/SCOPE_30.html (accessed December 14, 2010).

Stellman, J. M., S. D. Stellman, R. Christian, T. Weber, and C. Tomasallo. 2003. The extent and patterns of usage of Agent Orange and other herbicides in Vietnam. *Nature* 422(6933):681-687.

Still, K. R., D. P. Arfsten, W. W. Jederberg, L. V. Kane, and B. J. Larcom. 2003. Estimation of the health risks associated with polychlorinated biphenyl (PCB) concentrations found onboard older U.S. Navy vessels. *Applied Occupational and Environmental Hygiene* 18(10):737-758.

Young, A. L. 2009. *The history, use, disposition and environmental fate of Agent Orange*: New York, NY: Springer.

Young, A. L., P. E. Cecil, and J. F. Guilmartin. 2004a. Assessing possible exposures of ground troops to Agent Orange during the Vietnam war: The use of contemporary military records. *Environmental Science and Pollution Research* 11(6):349-358.

Young, A. L., J. P. Giesy, P. D. Jones, and M. Newton. 2004b. Environmental fate and bioavailability of Agent Orange and its associated dioxin during the Vietnam War. [Review] [82 refs]. *Environmental Science & Pollution Research* 11(6):359-370.

4

FATE AND TRANSPORT OF HERBICIDES USED IN VIETNAM

The potential for exposure of Blue Water Navy personnel to Agent Orange and its contaminant 2,3,7,8-tetrachlorodibenzo-p-dioxin (TCDD) is related to the fate of these chemicals in the Vietnamese environment. This chapter lays out the committee's understanding of the fate of Agent Orange after its environmental release as described in Chapter 3, with special attention to TCDD transport to and fate in coastal waters and atmospheric drift, and to modeling efforts to estimate environmental concentrations of TCDD. Because the relative importance of fate pathways is chemical specific, the discussion is restricted to TCDD that reached the environment through spraying and other releases of Agent Orange. The committee's rationale for the focus on TCDD is its understanding that TCDD is the toxic agent that has been associated with adverse health effects in Vietnam veterans (IOM, 1994).

The chapter takes a multimedia approach to discussing fate by looking at the air–vegetation–soil–water–sediment system of coastal Vietnam. Coastal fish are also included in the discussion. A multimedia approach considers all environmental compartments (such as air and soil) simultaneously, so intercompartmental transfers of TCDD are considered at the same time as the movement of TCDD within a single compartment. An example of a multimedia approach is consideration of TCDD evaporation from the surfaces of leaves to the air at the same time keeping in mind the movement of TCDD by means of air currents.

The committee did not identify any information on environmental concentrations of TCDD at the time of the Vietnam War that met current criteria for analytic quality assessment and quality control. The committee next considered using a mathematical model to estimate likely concentrations on the basis of TCDD that entered the environment. All models require a host of input parameter values, including standard physical and chemical properties of TCDD, characteristics of the

Vietnamese environment, and such chemical- and environment-specific parameter values as rates of TCDD degradation in Vietnamese coastal sediments. The committee found that, as is often the case for multimedia models and dioxins, input data and especially data with which to evaluate model performance were not available. Furthermore, large uncertainty would accompany any attempt to model overall TCDD fate by modeling emissions from individual spray paths on which data are available and scaling them up to hundreds of miles of coastline and coastal waters.

The committee explored the variability and uncertainty of several of the many parameters that could be used for assessing the fate and transport of TCDD in the environment, as described in the sections below. The goal of the exercise was a qualitative assessment of the fate of TCDD released during the Vietnam War. The discussion acknowledges the importance of location-specific factors that mediate chemical fate and transport, notably the tropical climate and the geography of Vietnam, which include episodic monsoons and the Mekong Delta, respectively. Most of the literature on the chemical fate of dioxins originates in temperate areas of the globe, such as Europe and North America, that differ substantially from the Vietnamese environment, and the committee was mindful of the differences as it developed its understanding of the fate of Agent Orange–associated TCDD in Vietnam.

THE VIETNAMESE ENVIRONMENT

The Republic of Vietnam is in the southern portion of the Indochina Peninsula in Southeast Asia. Its long, narrow shape extends nearly 1,100 km from north to south (about 8° to 17°N latitude) with a maximum width, in an east–west direction, of about 210 km and an area of nearly 170,000 km^2. About 1,400 km of the nearly 1,660 km of Vietnam's coastline is on the South China Sea, and the remaining (roughly 260 km) short stretch of coast on the southern end of the country faces the Gulf of Thailand. The inland portion of the northern two-thirds of southern Vietnam consists of high plateaus with coastal valleys and alluvial plains and streams that bring materials to the coastal zone. The coastline is irregular, with numerous headlands and bays.

The transport and fate of contaminants, such as TCDD, in the environment cannot be discussed without an understanding of the predominant hydrologic conditions of the area. The southern portion of

Vietnam is dominated by complex alluvial deltas, such as that of the Mekong River, and smaller river systems, such as that of the Bien Hoa. This portion of the country is mostly low lying and subject to frequent inundations and floods from monsoon rains; outside the monsoon season, river flows near the coast are controlled mainly by tidal forces. The coastline is mostly marshy and is lined with mangrove swamps distributed along much of the coastline in the Mekong Delta. It should be noted that the low-lying swamps at the interface between land and water were targets for heavy spraying of Agent Orange. Offshore of the swamps, the continental shelf off Vietnam slopes gently from the shoreline to the continental break at depths of about 100–200 m; from that point on, the slope is steeper, reaching depths of over 3,000 m in the South China Basin.

Climate of Vietnam

The Republic of Vietnam has a tropical monsoon climate with prevailing winds from the south to southeast during the summer monsoon and from the north to northeast during the winter monsoon. Air temperature and rainfall vary with the monsoon season. The average temperature and rainfall along the coast range from 24° to 30°C and from about 100 cm (40 in.) to over 300 cm (118 in.). The plateaus and higher foothills are cooler and have localized rainfall in excess of 400 cm (160 in.). The characteristics of the monsoon seasons (for example, winds, rainfall, and duration) vary throughout the country in that the winter monsoon (October–January) is more pronounced over the northern two-thirds of the country and the summer monsoon (May–August) tends to affect mostly the southern delta region.

The direction of predominant monsoonal winds follows the axis of the South China Sea, which gives the wind a maximum fetch that produces more powerful currents and larger waves during the fully developed monsoon season. At the beginning of the northeast monsoon (October), water in the South China Sea begins to flow to the southwest along the coast of Vietnam; it reaches its maximum, often exceeding 1 m/s, when the monsoon is fully developed (December). By April, the southerly flow intensity decreases with the decrease in monsoon intensity. The southwest or summer monsoon reverses the flow direction, and the surface water moves to the northeast, reaching its maximum flow in August.

Mekong River and Its Delta

The alluvial Mekong River is the dominant river system in southern Vietnam. Its estimated length is 4,350 km from its sources in southern China, it drains an area of 795,000 km^2, and it discharges 475 km^3 of water annually to the South China Sea. Hordoir et al. (2006) investigated river-coastal water flows of the Mekong Delta by developing a local coastal ocean model based on the Princeton Ocean Model of Blumberg and Mellor (1987). They ran the model for a year (1997) and evaluated it by comparing model simulations with conductivity–temperature–depth measurements made along the coast in March 1997 (the dry season) and at the beginning and end of October 1997 (the end of the monsoon season and the beginning of the dry season, respectively).

The results of Hordoir et al. (2006) indicated that although the flow from the Mekong Delta is very small compared with ocean currents, it influences ocean dynamics and physics in coastal regions as a result of the river's input of low-density fresh water into the higher-density saline water of the ocean. During winter, when the monsoons affect the northern part of the country, the total Mekong flow is about 2,500 m^3/s with the wind blowing predominantly from the northeast. That wind creates a compressed freshwater plume flowing southwest toward the Gulf of Thailand. The offshore plume, from the upper (Dai and Ham Luong) and lower (Dinh An, Tranh De, Hau, and Chieu) mouths of the Mekong Delta, would be well mixed vertically as a result of turbulence caused by the current's interaction with the shallow coastal shelf.

Hordoir et al. (2006) estimated that the offshore plume would be 5–10 m deep. The width of the plume would be 20–50 nautical miles (37–93 km) and be greatest off the southernmost point of the delta. During summer, when monsoons affect the south, the Mekong freshwater flow reaches a maximum of about 35,000 m^3/s with the wind changing radically from the northeast to the southwest. At that time, the winds cause the freshwater plume to head offshore, with only a weak current heading southeast. As a consequence, the freshwater influence would extend far offshore from the mouth of the delta. Hordoir et al. did their final simulation at the end of October, when the winds changed to the northeast and the river flow, although it decreased from early October, was still higher than that in winter; this resulted in a broader plume that hugged the coast and again flowed in a southeast direction.

FATE AND TRANSPORT OF AGENT ORANGE–ASSOCIATED TCDD IN THE VIETNAMESE ENVIRONMENT

As discussed in Chapter 3, 95% of the tactical herbicide used during the Vietnam War was applied by aerial spraying as part of Operation Ranch Hand (Stellman et al., 2003). Figure 4-1 illustrates the entry, transport, and fate pathways of Agent Orange–associated TCDD in the Vietnamese environment. The amount of TCDD that was sprayed in Vietnam during the Operation Ranch Hand missions has been variously estimated at 221–336 kg (Stellman et al., 2003) and 105–119 kg (Young, 2009). As described in Chapter 3, aerial applications of Agent Orange were conducted to deliver the maximum amount of herbicide to the forest canopy and to minimize spray drift.

An unknown fraction of aerial spraying occurred close to or over water—either rivers or coastal zones. Rivers were targeted because they served as transportation pathways. III Corps Area, north of the Mekong Delta, was the most heavily sprayed area of Vietnam (IOM, 1994). That area includes mangrove swamps and wetland soils, which, as described earlier, are organically rich and subject to seasonal inundation. Agent Orange could enter water courses by runoff from soil and vegetation from the sprayed areas. Agent Orange could also enter water courses from the spraying of river banks by the Brown Water Navy. The amount of Agent Orange applied to the river banks is uncertain, but it was less than 5% of the total amount used in Vietnam (Young, 2009). The committee assumed that most herbicide was released in air by aerial spraying (Figure 4-1[A]) and entered the water either by direct spraying over waterways or deposition of spray drift (Figure 4-1[9]) or indirectly by runoff from soil or vegetation (Figure 4-1[7]).

Modeling Fate and Transport of TCDD

The goal of assessing the fate and transport of Agent Orange–associated TCDD in the environment was to determine concentrations of TCDD that would probably have been found in each environmental compartment. On the basis of the presence or absence of TCDD, it might be possible to determine whether military personnel in Vietnam, particularly Blue Water Navy veterans, had the opportunity for exposure to TCDD and at what concentrations.

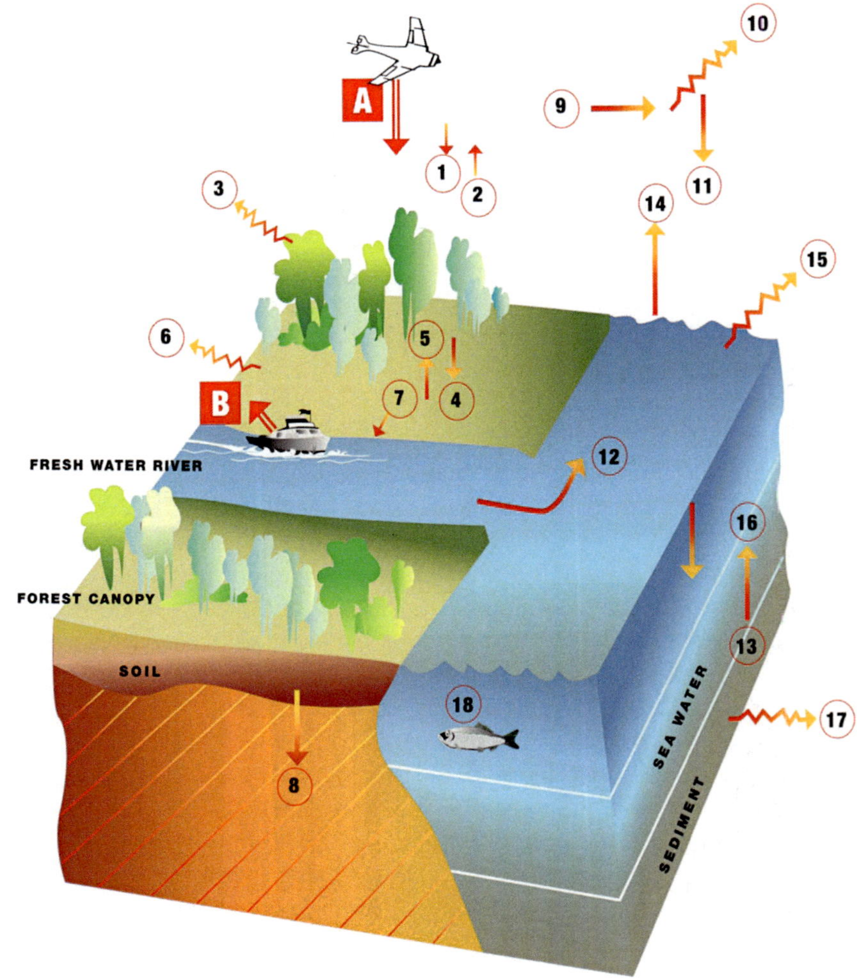

A. Aerial spray missions
B. Riverine spray missions

1. Deposition from air to forest canopy
2. Volatilization from forest canopy
3. Photodegradation on leaves
4. Deposition from forest to soils
5. Volatilization from soil to air
6. Degradation in soil due to microbial action, hydrolysis, and photolysis
7. Transport from soil to surface water, e.g. rivers and coastal waters
8. Leaching from soil to groundwater and groundwater discharge to surface waters
9. Spray drift and advective air flow of volatilized herbicide
10. Photodegradation in air
11. Atmospheric deposition to surface water
12. Advection of river discharge according to current
13. Deposition from water to sediment
14. Volatilization from water to air
15. Degradation in water column
16. Sediment resuspension
17. Degradation in sediment

FIGURE 4-1 Environmental fate and transport processes for Agent Orange and TCDD.

Mathematical models of chemical fate are widely used to reconstruct historical, current, and future conditions after an emission into a specified environment. A variety of models have been used to estimate the fate of polychlorinated dibenzodioxins and polychlorinated dibenzofurans (PCDDs and PCDFs), of which TCDD is one. Atmospheric dispersion models—such as TREND (van Jaarlsveld and Schutter, 1993), CMAQ (Zhang et al., 2009), and HYSPLIT (Cohen et al., 2002)—have been used to track PCDD and PCDF emissions over North America and Europe, where emissions originate mainly from combustion processes, such as municipal solid-waste incineration. There are three major constraints in using such models in the context of Agent Orange application in Vietnam. First, the models are extremely data intensive in that they require detailed information of time-dependent or statistically averaged meteorologic conditions (that is, historical weather data) at the time of chemical release. Such data were not available to the committee for simulating Vietnamese meteorologic conditions during the Vietnam War.

Second, the models have been applied to simulate PCDD and PCDF emissions from combustion in temperate regions. Translating the model to spray emissions in Vietnam requires detailed information on chemical partitioning and reaction rates in tropical regions. As explained below, there is a paucity of information on Vietnamese environmental conditions.

Third, the models must be evaluated with measured chemical concentrations, which could be another set of related compounds, such as polycyclic aromatic hydrocarbons. Model evaluation is crucial for gaining confidence that the model is providing reasonable representations of reality. Data on model evaluation specific to Vietnam are not available. This is a critical need because to the committee's knowledge such models have not been used to estimate the fate of Agent Orange in Vietnam, although there was some simulation of Agent Orange fate in tropical conditions at Elgin Air Force Base in Florida during the Vietnam War (Young, 2009).

Multimedia box models have also been used to estimate "average" TCDD fate and concentrations in the environmental compartments of air, water, soil, sediment, and fish. The models emphasize chemical transport among environmental compartments but simplify movement within each compartment, such as air and water. *Box* refers to the assumption that each compartment is a well-mixed box rather than having detailed spatial resolution, as in the air-dispersion models discussed above. Examples of the application of multimedia models to dioxins are the single box model of Dalla Valle et al. (2003) and the multibox models of Persson et al. (2006) and Sommerfreund et al. (2010). These models have the same constraints as the air-dispersion models but do not require the same level of detailed knowledge of time-dependent meteorology and hydrodynamics.

Models like AgDISP and AgDRIFT have been developed to estimate near-field (within about 1 km) deposition and drift of pesticides applied by aerial spraying. AgDISP and AgDRIFT consider climate (for example, temperature and relative humidity) and spray conditions but not other facets of fate, such as atmospheric degradation or multimedia transfer (Bilanin et al., 1989; Bird et al., 2002; Teske et al., 2002).

The committee concluded that using models to estimate likely concentrations of TCDD in the Vietnamese environment to which Blue Water Navy personnel would be exposed is not possible because of the lack of data with which to assign values to model parameters. Even if parameter values could be assigned, data are not available to evaluate model performance. In the absence of model evaluation, the uncertainty of model results would be too large for the committee to be confident that they were reasonable. Thus, the committee turned to understanding the fate of TCDD on a qualitative or descriptive basis.

Transport of TCDD in the Environment[1]

The committee considered the fate pathways of Agent Orange and TCDD after its environmental release from aerial spraying (Figure 4-1[A]) and riverbank spraying (Figure 4-1[B]). Although the committee believes that all important fate processes are discussed, the fraction of Agent Orange subject to one or another is highly uncertain. The following discussion is therefore qualitative, not quantitative, and does not include any estimate of likely environmental concentrations of TCDD that prevailed during the Vietnam War. Rather, the purpose of the following discussion is to evaluate qualitatively the likelihood that TCDD concentrations in the Vietnamese air and water after Agent Orange spraying would exceed the TCDD concentrations that would be expected in the absence of Agent Orange spraying.

---

[1]The discussion in this section refers to the letters and numbers in Figure 4-1.

TCDD Fate in the Atmosphere

Spray drift

Spray sorties were timed to coincide with calm days and occurred very early in the morning to maximize the contact of herbicide with the forest and to minimize spray drift. Young (2009) summarized calculations of the fate of Agent Orange sprayed in Operation Ranch Hand sorties. Young assumed an atmospheric deposition velocity of 30 cm/s^2 for Agent Orange on the basis of a minimum droplet size of <100 μm in the spray emitted from the spray nozzles on the C-123 aircraft. He reported that that would mean that 87% of the Agent Orange sprayed would reach the forest canopy and the remaining 13% would be subject to spray drift with an exponential dropoff in drift as a function of perpendicular distance from the line of spraying.

The Institute of Medicine (IOM) Committee on Making Best Use of the Agent Orange Exposure Reconstruction Model (IOM, 2008) reported various distances that Agent Orange spray could drift, from 2 km (Darrow, 1969) to more than 10 km (Department of the Army, 1971). Ginevan et al. (2009a), however, stated that less than 2% drift would have occurred on the basis of simulations of the AgDRIFT pesticide-spray model. Ross and Ginevan (2007) arrived at an area subject to herbicide deposition of less than 1/40 that of the Stellman model (Stellman and Stellman, 2004).

At issue with the varied estimates of the distance over which spray drift would have occurred is the amount of herbicide deposited on land or water (Figure 4-1[1, 11]). All assume that deposition would drop off exponentially with distance from the spray path, that is, deposition would be greatest at the edge of the spray path. The committee asked the US Department of Agriculture's Agricultural Research Service to run simulations of the AgDISP pesticide-spray model (Clint Hoffman, USDA ARS, personal communication, December 27, 2010) to evaluate that assumption. With a range of input values intended to reproduce conditions during Agent Orange spraying and drift over open water—for example, 46–76 m release height, 1–6.2 m/s wind speed, 25–30°C, 90% relative humidity, stable atmospheric conditions, ASAE medium–coarse droplet distribution, and 25 L/ha spray volume rate—the AGDISP model estimated that more than 90% of the Agent Orange sprayed was deposited within 100–200 m of the spray path when it was sprayed from a height of 46 and 76 m, respectively. However, a wind of 6.2 m/s, or about 12 knots, the maximum at which spray missions were conducted, could increase the spray drift so that 90–95% of the amount sprayed would be deposited within 800 m of the spray path (Clint Hoffman, US Department of Agriculture, Agricultural Research Service, personal communication, December 30, 2010). According to runs of AgDISP over a forest canopy versus water, the committee expects that drift would be greater over water than over land because the smoothness of the water surface maximizes drift.

Conditions favoring spray drift from coast to land would occur during the day, particularly during spring and early summer, when the land temperature would exceed that of the coastal waters. That phenomenon can be explained by the land heating faster than water, which causes the air over the land to become warmer and less dense. As the air rises, it is replaced by cooler, denser air flowing in from over the water. That causes an onshore wind, called a sea breeze. At night, the land cools faster than water, as does the corresponding air; the warmer air over the water rises and is replaced by the cooler, denser air from the land, creating an offshore wind called a land breeze. Most sorties were flown early in the morning, when a sea breeze was expected. Thus, the daily timing of the sorties favored sea-breeze conditions, which would minimize spray drift over coastal waters.

Atmospheric fate

The 13% of the Agent Orange not deposited on the forest canopy would be subject to spray drift (Figure 4-1[9]) (Young 2009). The committee considered direct aerial spraying over water. While airborne in Agent Orange spray, TCDD would partition between gas and particle phases. The fraction in the gas phase in temperate urban environments relative to total TCDD has been estimated to vary from 20% to nearly 90% (for example, 10–80% would be sorbed by particles) (Bidleman, 1988; Eitzer and Hites 1989a,b; Hippelein et al., 1996). Gas-phase TCDD in air would degrade by reaction with hydroxyl radicals and to a lesser extent photodegradation (degradation of a molecule due to ultraviolet radiation) (Figure 4-1[10]) (Atkinson et al., 1987).

Degradation of particle-sorbed TCDD is negligible (Koester and Hites, 1992). Podoll et al. (1986) calculated an upper limit for a photolytic half-life of 58 minutes for TCDD in the vapor phase at 40°N latitude. Atkinson et al. (1987) estimated, through an analysis of literature values and by chemical analogy, that the half-life of gas-phase TCDD would be about 3 days (assuming 12 h of sunlight and average global hydroxyl radical concentration of 1.5×10^6 molecules/cm^3). Cohen et al. (2002) mathematically derived a half-life of TCDD due to reaction with OH radicals of 5 days, on the basis of the same assumptions as those of Atkinson et al. Cohen et al. assumed a photodegradation half-life of 2 days on the basis of a review of the literature. Katritzky et al. (2010) calculated a photodegradation half-life for TCDD of 55.5–72.3 h, or 2.3–3 days. These half-lives are long enough to minimize the importance of atmospheric degradation relative to spray drift and deposition.

Deposition on the intentionally targeted vegetation would occur, along with some on soil and surface water, as discussed below (Figure 4-1[11]). Because most spraying occurred during calm conditions with no precipitation, it is assumed that most atmospheric deposition would be dry deposition. Other mechanisms that would deliver TCDD to the coastal surface water would be gas-phase absorption due to diffusion, assuming that the concentration (or more correctly fugacity or activity) gradient was from air to water. Wet deposition or washout due to gas-phase and particle-phase washout is considered the least likely of the deposition mechanisms because most spraying occurred during dry conditions; however, washout would be an efficient mechanism for removing TCDD and other compounds from air. Thus, the committee concluded that with atmospheric deposition, there was an opportunity for herbicides applied by aerial spraying in Vietnam to enter inland waters of Vietnam and the coastal waters that received the discharge from those waters in addition to herbicide that was applied directly to water.

Deposition of TCDD from Air onto Forest Canopy

Young et al. (2004) conducted a detailed analysis of the fate of Agent Orange, and TCDD in particular, sprayed over the Vietnamese forests during the war. They reported results of tests at Elgin Air Force Base in Florida that were designed to simulate environmental conditions during Operation Ranch Hand. They estimated that 87% of the herbicide would have reached the tree canopy within 1 min within or near the spray swath (Figure 4-1[1]). That estimate assumed a leaf area index (LAI) of 5; that is, the area of leaves was 5 times greater than the area of the ground surface below. They further stated that 99% of the sprayed Agent Orange would affect the forest if sorption by tree branches and trunks and the vegetative understory were included. No other studies were found that estimated the amount of TCDD deposited on target spray areas versus the amount subject to atmospheric drift under conditions relevant to the Vietnamese situation.

At the leaf surface, TCDD would contact and sorb to the waxy cuticle of leaves. McCrady and Maggard (1993) measured an initial uptake rate constant of 1,750 h^{-1} for TCDD, or an uptake half-life of 1.4 s. The committee was unable to assess the validity of those results, which were reported as an average of several experiments. It is possible that the uptake rate was inflated (that is, too fast) because of uptake by walls of the experimental chamber, which would reduce the concentration of TCDD in chamber air. Young et al. (2004) commented that TCDD sorbed by the leaf cuticle "could not be physically dislodged." However, other studies have shown that the finger-like protrusions of the cuticle, with sorbed contaminants, can be eroded from leaf surfaces; this can lead to transport of sorbed contaminants from the leaf and possibly to deposition on soil (Sauter et al., 1987; Turunen and Hattunen, 1991).

Loss of TCDD from Vegetation

A fraction of TCDD that came into contact with the leaf would be expected to evaporate (volatilize) as air temperatures increased during the day after spraying (Figure 4-1[2]). A low but measurable rate of volatilization of TCDD from foliage would be expected because of its low vapor pressure (2.0×10^{-7} Pa at 25°C). Temperature-dependent volatilization of persistent semivolatile chemicals from vegetation has been documented in temperate zones (Hornbuckle and Eisenreich, 1996; Su et al., 2007), but that phenomenon has not been reliably measured for dioxins (Lohmann and Jones, 1998). Bacci et al. (1992) found that 1,2,3,4-TCDD, which has partitioning properties similar to that of 2,3,7,8-TCDD, has a strong leaf/air equilibrium bioconcentration factor of 1.03×10^{8}, suggesting that TCDD will move from the vapor phase in air to leaf surfaces. TCDD on leaf surfaces could also be lost via photodegradation (Figure 4-1[3]) with estimated half-lives around 3–6 h (Crosby and Wong, 1977; Choudhry and Webster, 1989; Schuler et al., 1998). Crobsy and Wong (1977) measured the rate of photodegradation of Agent Orange that contained TCDD at 15 ppm applied to excised leaves of a rubber plant when exposed to sunlight for a half life of about 2 h. They measured a slower photodegradation rate (half life of about 5–6 h) when Agent Orange was applied to glass plates; dark controls were unaffected. This suggests that photochemical dechlorination is a primary removal process for TCDD on leaf surfaces. McCrady and Maggard (1993) reported a much longer TCDD half-life of 44 days via photodegradation measured during a sophisticated chamber experiment in which grass was exposed to gas-phase radiolabeled TCDD and then illuminated by lamps intended to simulate natural sunlight. The temperatures in the chamber ranged from 18° to 28°C. The authors found that the volatilization half-life was greater than 128 h, which led them to conclude that photodegradation was the main mechanism of loss of TCDD from grass. They commented that the shorter photodegradation half-life measured by Crosby and Wong could be attributable to the promotion of photodegradation by the other organic solvents in Agent Orange in contrast with the pure TCDD used in their experiment. On the basis of those studies, the committee concludes that the photodegradation half-life of TCDD delivered to foliage in Agent Orange would be hours to days, or even weeks, if leaves did not receive direct sunlight. It is also important to note that most experiments and calculations of photodegradation are conducted to simulate environmental conditions at about 40°N latitude; at this latitude, ultraviolet radiation from the sun is less intense than that at 16°N latitude, where Vietnam is.

Deposition of TCDD from Canopy to Soil

TCDD could deposit on soil directly from Agent Orange spraying, by the falling of sprayed foliage, by dry deposition of eroded leaf waxes, and by leaf washoff during precipitation (Figure 4-1[4]). Ginevan et al. (2009a) cited results from the AgDRIFT model that indicated that 1–2% of Agent Orange sprayed aerially would reach the ground. Several researchers (Horstmann et al., 1997; Brorstrom-Lunden and Lofgren, 1998; Wania and McLachlan, 2001) have documented higher concentrations of dioxins in forest than in pasture soils as a result of leaf accumulation of atmospheric dioxins at ambient concentrations and later transfer from plant to soil via the deposition mechanisms mentioned above. In other words, the tree canopy is efficient in collecting atmospherically deposited dioxin and transferring it to soil in cases in which dioxins or other herbicides have not caused leaf dieback. Dioxin transfer to soils from the tree canopy has not been assessed where TCDD was a component of a herbicide.

TCDD Fate in Soil

The organic content of most Vietnamese soils ranges between 1.8% and 5% (Ton, 1996). Because of TCDD's hydrophobicity (a chemical's tendency to partition to water and seek nonpolar media, such as soil organic matter), those soils would be efficient sinks for TCDD. Dioxins, in general, are known to be highly persistent in soils (Wania and McLachlan, 2000), as confirmed by Freeman and Schroy (1986), who found TCDD in soils some 12 years after a field experiment at Elgin Air Force Base that involved applying Agent Orange to soils at a depth of 10 cm. In general, the small fraction of TCDD not sorbed to soil would be lost through volatilization (Figure 4-1[5]). In an experiment at Times Beach, Missouri, where TCDD-contaminated oil had been applied to roads in the early 1970s, Freeman and Schroy (1989) found that volatilization of TCDD from the soil column was very slow with a flux of 6×10^{-8} kg/d m^2. In 1984, the observed loss of TCDD from the top 3 mm of soil was 50%; 0.1% of the TCDD in the top 1 mm of soil was estimated to be lost by volatilization, with the remaining TCDD lost by photodegradation. Virtually no TCDD was lost from the soil below this depth. Muir et al. (1985) concluded that the loss of radiolabeled 1,3,6,8-TCDD applied to field soil resulted in a half-life of 131–321 days and could have been due primarily to volatilization. The half-life in sediments was greater than 600 days. Although not large, rates of volatilization would be expected to increase after defoliation when more sunlight would reach soils and soil temperatures would increase.

TCDD in soils may be degraded by microbial activity, hydrolysis, or sunlight (Figure 4-1[6]). Defoliation would also promote photodegradation in soils. Podoll et al. (1986) calculated that—based on TCDD's low Henry's constant of 12 torr M^{-1} and high octanol/water partition coefficient (K_{ow}) of approximately 3×10^8—in wet soil (1% organic carbon and 30% water by volume), 99.99% of the TCDD will be sorbed on soil and would not volatilize. However, in dry soil, TCDD would be subject to some volatilization but substantial TCDD would remain sorbed to the soil. Miller et al. (1989) found that direct photodegradation was important only at soil depths of less than 0.2 mm, so it would account for little of the total TCDD loss from soil. Young (1983) reported that 99.9% of the TCDD applied in herbicides at Elgin Air Force Base in Florida was photodegraded during and immediately after application. Crosby and Wong (1977) found slow but measurable loss of TCDD from soil surfaces exposed to direct sunlight.

Microbial degradation is expected to occur but over time scales of decades or even a century (Sinkkonen and Paasivirta, 2000), although these estimates pertain to temperate regions where microbial degradation is much slower than in warmer regions, such as Vietnam. Karch et al. (2004) note that microbial degradation of TCDD may be enhanced by the presence of herbicide which stimulates microbial activity.

Although the most likely fate of TCDD in soils is to remain in place for decades, a small amount may also be lost as a result of wind or rain erosion (Muir et al., 1985) and leaching to lower soil horizons (Freeman and Schroy, 1986) (Figure 4-1[7]). A very small amount of TCDD may leach from soil to shallow groundwater (Figure 4-1[8]). The most mobile fraction of TCDD would be associated with colloidal humic or organic material (also referred to as colloidal material in the literature). In contrast to the relatively immobile soil particles, colloids can sometimes travel and facilitate the transport of hydrophobic contaminants. However, colloid concentrations are usually extremely low because aquifers filter out colloids efficiently. Thus, it is highly unlikely that TCDD will have been relocated via groundwater colloids to the river water.

Especially during the flooding of coastal areas, erosion and leaching rather than volatilization followed by redeposition would be expected to deliver the greatest fraction of TCDD from soils to surface waters (Quinh et al., 1989). Erosion could be wind driven or water driven, and erosion rates would increase as defoliation proceeded.

The proximity of soils to waterways and the frequent flooding of the soils, particularly in the heavily sprayed III Corps Area, would increase the probability that soil-bound and humic-material-bound herbicides would reach water courses. The monsoon rains would be expected to transport the humic-bound and soil-bound herbicides to surface waters. Although it is logical to conclude that some fraction of TCDD and other herbicides applied in heavily sprayed areas would reach inland and coastal waters from soils, particularly as the forest is denuded, the amount of TCDD that entered water courses would be subject to enormous dilution from river flows. Quinh et al. (1989) report that the annual discharges of the Tien Giang and Hau Giang rivers in the Mekong Delta, are 92,000 m^3/s and 90,000 m^3/s, respectively, or "76% and 79% of their flows during the wet season."

Fate of TCDD in River Waters

If Agent Orange reached water, TCDD would be subject to photolysis. Podoll et al. (1986) estimated that the half-life of TCDD in near surface waters at 40° latitude in sunlight during the summer would be 21 hours compared with 118 hours in the winter. Photolysis would be hindered by the presence of sediment; because of its low water solubility, 0.0193 μg/L, TCDD would tend to sorb to suspended particles and humic material in the receiving waters (Hsieh et al., 1994) and hydrophobic nature. TCDD sorption to suspended particles and humic material would be highly likely in the turbid and humic-rich waters of the rivers in Vietnam. River-water quality is controlled largely by land-based runoff that, in turn, is controlled by precipitation. The committee was unable to obtain data related to water quality of rivers in Vietnam. It was presumed that the rivers carried organic matter, including humic material, from a terrestrial origin, possibly with sorbed TCDD. On reaching estuaries at river mouths along the coast, particles, colloidal organic matter, and sorbed TCDD would be subject to flocculation and agglomeration as colloids bind to one another and to particles. That creates a zone of high turbidity (a maximum-turbidity zone) that can act as a partial filter for the removal or immobilization of sorbed TCDD from the water column. The mechanism will be less efficient in removing dissolved TCDD, which would be expected to occur at minuscule concentrations (Geyer et al., 2004). The efficiency of the maximum-turbidity zone depends on the concentration of suspended sediment, organic carbon content, and the estuarine chemistry and flow regime. Away from the estuarine and coastal regions, marine water becomes more homogeneous over a wider area, although patchiness due to a lack of mixing occurs. Thus, the committee concluded that whereas most particle-bound and colloid-bound TCDD would deposit in the estuaries of river deltas, some small fraction of total TCDD in the dissolved phase or bound to colloids and particles would make its way out to coastal waters.

Fate of TCDD in Marine Coastal Waters

As TCDD entered the coastal waters of Vietnam as a result of spray drift and atmospheric deposition (Figure 4-1[A]), direct spraying on and along rivers (Figure 4-1[B]), and river discharge, it would be in three phases: truly dissolved, sorbed to humic material (colloidal), and particle bound. Humic-material-bound and particle-bound TCDD would have a high probability of settling to the sediments in estuaries as the fresh river water meets the saline coastal water, as discussed above. A fraction of TCDD that reached coastal waters would be transported by the prevailing coastal zone currents, as described by Hordoir et al. (2006) (Figure 4-1[12]). Although the committee cannot estimate the concentration, the TCDD that entered the water (that is, the TCCD load) would be expected to be greatly diluted at this stage, and dilution would increase with distance from shore.

TCDD could be lost from the top 1–5 m of coastal waters by photodegradation (Figure 4-1[15]). Photodegradation could be important in this top layer of water, presuming that the waters were not excessively turbid; humic material and particles discharged to the coastal marine waters from rivers reduce photodegradation as a result of shading.

Reported half-life values for TCDD in surface water range from 4–5 days (Dulin et al., 1986) in the summer at 40°N latitude and 25°C to up to 600 days (Ward and Matsumura, 1978) at 24°C using water from Lake Mendota and Lake Wingra in Wisconsin. It is expected that the half-life of TCCD in Vietnamese coastal waters, if they were relatively clear, would be shorter than that because of the higher intensity of ultraviolet radiation hitting Vietnamese water than that at 40°N. Hydrolysis is not expected to be an important degradation process for TCDD (Sinkkonen and Paasivirta, 2000).

In most waters, the greatest fraction of TCDD would bind to particles such as algae, detritus, and mineral matter, because these particles are typically most abundant, followed by binding to humic material; finally, a very small fraction of TCDD would be truly dissolved in water, as mentioned above. The partitioning of TCDD among those three would be a function of the concentrations of particles and humic material in coastal waters. The committee was unable to identify information on the concentrations of particles and humic material in Vietnamese coastal waters. Particle-sorbed TCDD would be lost from the water column to bottom sediment by deposition (Figure 4-1[13]). The loss rate would be determined by the concentration of particles and their settling rate. Humic-bound TCDD would be transported by water movement and diffusive exchange with sediment but not deposition, because humic colloids are not subject to settling. Diffusive exchange of colloidal TCDD is not expected to be an important loss process (Sommerfreund et al., 2010). Volatilization of truly dissolved TCDD (Figure 4-1[14]) is also expected to be minimal because of the negligible fraction of TCDD that would be in this phase and the low vapor pressure of TCDD.

TCDD sorbed to coastal sediment particles could return to the water column as a result of sediment resuspension (Figure 4-1[16]). A smaller amount could return to the water column as a result of sediment-to-water diffusion of colloidal TCDD; however, this is usually negligible (Sommerfreund et al., 2010). Resuspension of sediment-sorbed chemicals can be an important process in shallow waters, such as the coastal zone off the Mekong Delta, where the sea bottom drops from a depth of 5 m extending about 5 km offshore to 20 m about 40 km offshore (Hordoir et al., 2006). Resuspension events in shallow waters are expected when winds are high, at times of very high river discharge (for example, during the summer monsoon season) when turbulent flows could entrain sediment particles, and possibly as a result of a ship dropping or pulling up an anchor. Although resuspension can bring particle-bound chemicals back into the water column, they will redeposit as the turbulence dissipates. Thus, sediment-bound chemicals can cycle between sediment and the water column.

The final loss processes, which ultimately remove TCDD from the aquatic system, are microbial degradation in sediment and burial in deeper sediment (Figure 4-1[17]). As is the case with soils, degradation by anaerobic microorganisms in sediment is expected over time scales of 10s to 100s of years (Sinkkonen and Paasivirta, 2000).

LIMITATIONS OF AND UNCERTAINTIES ON FATE AND TRANSPORT OF TCDD

No studies of the fate of Agent Orange or TCDD in the Vietnamese environment at the time of the Vietnam War were found. As noted in the discussion above, the committee's conclusions are based on a theoretical understanding of fate processes of TCDD. Field studies of TCDD have been undertaken in temperate zones or with systems set up to simulate conditions that prevailed during the Vietnam War, such as the experiments conducted at Elgin Air Force Base in Florida. Modeling results cited here, such as those of AgDRIFT and AgDISP, are based on conditions similar to those in the Vietnam War.

The several studies below have reported measurable TCDD in environmental samples taken in Vietnam and Laos from the 1980s onward that are attributed to the use of Agent Orange during the Vietnam War. Those studies indicate that TCDD accumulated at low concentrations in aquatic systems (e.g., Pavlov et al., 2004) or soils, and this suggests transport from sprayed regions or substantial TCDD degradation since Operation Ranch Hand. The results of the earlier studies are confounded by issues of TCDD detection; however, analytic methods have improved dramatically over the last few decades. TCDD contamination has been found around areas known to have been used as Agent Orange depots. Schecter et al. (1989a,b) analyzed five samples of river silt taken from the Dong Nai River (upstream of Ho Chi Minh City [Saigon] and near a village that had been heavily sprayed with Agent Orange) and one sample from the Saigon River in the Ho Chi Minh City area in 1985 and 1986 using a high-resolution analytic method. They found that TCDD in sediment samples from the Dong Nai River were below the limit of detection (21 pg/g dry weight), however, TCDD was present at 210 pg/g in sediment (limit of detection, 6 pg/g dry weight) from the Saigon River in Ho Chi Minh City. The latter finding is for only one sample. In 1999, Schecter et al. (2001) measured concentrations of TCDD in soil and sediment samples taken from Bien Hoa Air Base and its vicinity in southern Vietnam and from Hanoi. Concentrations were 1,164,699 pg/g (ppt) dry matter in soil from the air base where Agent Orange was known to be used, stored, and spilled; 0.8–117 ng/kg (ppt) in sediments of Bien Hung Lake near the air base; and 0.8–1.5 ng/kg in the Dong Nai River that flows from the lake; no TCDD was detected in the sediments of the Hanoi River. More recently, Piazza et al. (2007) reported low concentrations of total dioxins and furans, particularly TCDD, in the sediment of Vietnamese coastal lagoons and some inland waters. That observation led them to conclude that degradation took place shortly after Agent Orange was sprayed. Dwernychuk et al. (2002) found increased concentrations of TCDD in soil and food samples systematically collected in 1996–1999 from areas of the Aluoi Valley in Vietnam known to have been heavily sprayed with Agent Orange compared with areas that received less spraying. The highest concentrations were found in soil and animal fat collected in a Vietnamese village on a former US Army base where Agent Orange had been stored during 1963–1966. Nhu et al. (2009) also found that TCDD concentrations in soil and breast-milk samples taken from Agent Orange-sprayed areas of Vietnam in 2002–2003 were higher than those in samples from nonsprayed areas. In addition, Quinh et al. (1989) suggested that the relatively high concentrations of TCDD found in adipose tissue of some Vietnamese residents of areas that had not been heavily sprayed with Agent Orange might be caused by the runoff of TCDD-contaminated soils from sprayed areas into rivers during the monsoon season with subsequent flooding carrying the contaminated soil into fields.

CONCLUSIONS

The committee reviewed the fate of Agent Orange and TCDD in particular in the Vietnamese environment as a result of spray applications during the Vietnam War. The discussion is entirely qualitative because the committee was not able to quantify any component of the fate processes discussed. Furthermore, insufficient data were available even to attempt a rudimentary calculation of the fate of TCDD emitted into the Vietnamese environment during the war.

On the basis of a review of the literature and knowledge of fate and transport processes in the context of Vietnam, the committee concludes that most Agent Orange and TCDD sprayed as part of Operation Ranch Hand intercepted target vegetation. Undoubtedly, some fraction entered soil either immediately after spraying or as the vegetation died back because of Agent Orange's herbicidal activity. Most TCDD deposited on soil would be expected to persist, as has been confirmed by some more recent studies of contemporary dioxin concentrations in soils (Dwernychuk et al., 2002) but not other earlier studies (Schecter et al., 1989). The committee concludes that Agent Orange and TCDD could have entered rivers from spraying along riverbanks (although this was a small fraction of the total Agent Orange applied in Vietnam) or from soil runoff, particularly in heavily sprayed areas that experienced frequent flooding. River loading would be highly diluted by river flows. A substantial fraction of particles and humic material to which TCDD would be bound would settle in river mouths and estuaries because of estuarine dynamics and chemistry, although it is puzzling that recent studies have found minimal residual TCDD in sediment dated back to Agent Orange spraying during the war.

TCDD would enter coastal marine water from river discharge (albeit a very small load because of the mechanisms discussed) and from spray drift. The committee concludes that TCDD loading due to spray drift could have occurred but would have been minimal. Atmospheric deposition of TCDD on coastal waters from spray drift would have been greatly diluted in these waters. Given the paucity of information and the variability and uncertainty in the available information, the committee concludes that it is not possible to estimate the likely concentrations of TCDD in marine waters and air at the time of the Vietnam War.

REFERENCES

Atkinson, R. 1987. Estimation of OH radical reaction rate constants and atmospheric lifetimes for polychlorobiphenyls, dibenzo-p-dioxins, and dibenzofurans. *Environmental Science and Technology* 21:305-307.

Bacci, E., M. J. Cerejeira, C. Gaggi, G. Chemello, D. Calamari, and M. Vighi. 1992. Chlorinated dioxins: Volatilization from soils and bioconcentration in plant leaves. *Bulletin of Environmental Contamination and Toxicology* 48:401-408.

Bidleman, T. F. 1988. Atmospheric processes: Wet and dry deposition of organic compounds are controlled by their vapor-particle partitioning. *Environmental Science and Technology* 22:361-367.

Bilanin, A. J., M. E. Teske, B. W. Barry, and R. B. Ekbald.1989. AGDISP: The aircraft spray dispersion model, code development, and experimental validation. *Transactions of the ASAE* 32(1):327-334.

Bird, S. L., S. G. Perry, S. L. Ray, and M. E. Teske. 2002. Evaluation of the AGDISP aerial spray algorithms in the AgDRIFT model. Environmental Toxicology and Chemistry 21(3):672-681.

Blumberg, A. F., and G. L. Mellor. 1987. A description of a three-dimensional coastal ocean circulation model. In *Three-Dimensional Coastal Ocean Models*, Vol. 4, edited by N. Heaps. Washington, DC: American Geophysical Union.

Brorstrom-Lunden, E., and C. Lofgren. 1998. Atmospheric fluxes of persistent semivolatile organic pollutants to a forest ecological system at the Swedish west coast and accumulation in spruce needles. *Environmental Pollution* 102(139-149):277-291.

Choudhry, G. G., and G. R. B. Webster. 1989. Environmental photochemistry of PCDDs quantum yields of the direct phototransformation of 1,2,3,7-tetra-, 1,3,6,8-tetra, 1,2,3,4,6,7,8-hepta, and 1,2,3,4,6,7,8,9-octachlorodibenzo-p-dioxin in aqueous acetonitrile and their sunlight half-lives. *Journal of Agricultural and Food Chemistry* 37(1):254-261.

Cohen, M., et al. 2002. Modeling the Atmospheric Transport and Deposition of PCDD/F to the Great Lakes. *Journal of Environmental Science and Technology* 36:4831-4845.

Crosby, D. G., and A. S. Wong. 1977. Environmental degradation of 2,3,7,8-tetrachlorodibenzo-p-dioxin (TCDD). *Science* 195:1337-1338.

Dalla Valle, A. 2004. The skew-normal distribution. In *Skew Elliptical Distributions and Their Applications*, edited by M.G. Genton. Boca Raton, FL: CRC Press. Pp. 2-24.

Darrow, R. A. 1969. *Report of trip to Republic of Vietnam, 15 August-2 September 1969*. Department of the Army.

Department of the Army. 1971. *Field manual: Tactical employment of herbicides*. Washington, DC: Headquarters.

Dulin, D., H. Drossman, and T. Mill. 1986. Products and quantum yields for photolysis of chromoaromatics in water. *Environmental Science and Technology* 20:72-77.

Dwernychuk, L. W., H. D. Cau, C. T Hatfield, T. G. Boivin, T. M. Hung, P. T. Dung, and N. D. Thai. 2002. Dioxin reservoirs in southern Viet Nam—A legacy of Agent Orange. *Chemosphere* 47:117-137.

Eitzer, B. D., and R. A. Hites. 1989a. Atmospheric transport and deposition of polychlorinated dibenzo p-dioxins and dibenzofurans. *Environmental Science and Technology* 1989:1396-1401.

Eitzer, B. D., and R. A. Hites. 1989b. Polychlorinated dibenzo-p-dioxins and dibenzofurans in the ambient atmosphere of Bloomington, Indiana. *Environmental Science and Technology* 23:1389-1395.

EPA (Environmental Protection Agency). 1993. *Interim report on data and methods for assessment of 2,3,7,8-tetrachlorodibenzo-p-dioxin risks to aquatic life and associated wildlife.* Washington, DC: Office of Water.

Freeman, R. A., and J. M. Schroy. 1986. Modeling the transport of 2,3,7,8-TCDD and other low volatility chemicals in soils. *Environmental Progress* 5(1).

Geyer, W. R., P. S. Hill, and G. C. Kineke. 2004. The transport, transformation and dispersal of sediment by buoyant coastal flows. *Continental Shelf Research* 24(7-8):927-949.

Ginevan, M. E., J. H. Ross, and D. K. Watkins. 2009. Assessing exposure to allied ground troops in the Vietnam War: A comparison of AgDRIFT and Exposure Opportunity Index models. *Journal of Exposure Science and Environmental Epidemiology* 19(2):187-200.

Hippelein, M., H. Kaupp, G. Dorr, M. S. McLauchan, and O. Hutzinger. 1996. Baseline contamination assessment for a new resource recovery facility in Germany. Part II: Atmospheric concentration of PCDD/F. *Chemosphere* 32:1605-1616.

Hordoir, R., K. D. Nguyen, and J. Polcher. 2006. Simulating tropical river plumes, a set of parameterizations based on macroscale data: A test case in the Mekong Delta region. *Journal of Geophysical Research-Oceans* 111(C9).

Hornbuckle, K. C., and S. J. Eisenreich. 1996. Dynamics of gaseous semivolatile organic compounds in a terrestrial ecosystem—Effects of diurnal and seasonal climate variations. *Atmospheric Environment* 30:3935-3945.

Hsieh, D. P. H., F. F. Chiao, R. C. Currie, and T. E. McKone. 1994. *Intermedia transfer factors for contaminants found at hazardous waste sites: 2,3,7,8-tetrachlorodibenzo-p-dioxin (TCDD). Final draft report.* Davis, CA: University of California, Department of Environmental Toxicology.

IOM (Institute of Medicine). 1994. *Veterans and Agent Orange: Health effects of herbicides used in Vietnam.* Washington, DC: National Academy Press.

IOM. 2008. *The utility of proximity-based herbicide exposure assessment in epidemiologic studies of Vietnam veterans.* Washington, DC: The National Academies Press.

Karch, N. J., D. K. Watkins, A. L. Young, and M. E. Ginevan. 2004. Environmental fate of TCDD and Agent Orange and bioavailability to troops in Vietnam. *Organohalogen Compounds* 66:3689-3694.

Katritzky, A. R., S. H. Slavov, I. B. Stoyanova-Slavova, and M. Karelson. 2010. Correlation of the photolysis half-lives of polychlorinated dibenzo-p-dioxins and dibenzofurans with molecular structure. *Journal of Physical Chemistry* 114:2684-2688.

Koester, C. J., and R. A. Hites. 1992. Photodegradation of polychlorinated dioxins and dibenzofurans adsorbed to fly-ash. *Environmental Science & Technology* 26(3):502-507.

Lohmann, R., and K. C. Jones. 1998. Dioxins and furans in air and deposition: A review of levels, behaviour and processes. *Science of the Total Environment* 219(1):53-81.

McGrady, J. K., and S. P. Maggard. 1993. Uptake and photodegradation of 2,3,7,8-tetrachlorodibenzo-p-dioxin sorbed to grass foliage. *Environmental Science and Technology* 27:343-350.

Miller, G. C., V. R. Hebert, M. J. Miille, R. Mitzel, and R. G. Zepp, R.G. 1989. Photolysis of octachlorodibenzo-p-dioxin on soils: production of 2,3,7,8-TCDD. *Chemosphere* 18:1265-1274.

Muir, D. C. G., A. L. Yarechewski, R. L. Corbet, G. R. B. Webster, and A. E. Smith. 1985. Laboratory and field studies on the fate of 1,3,6,8-tetrachlorodibenzo-p-dioxin in soil and sediments. *Journal of Agricultural and Food Chemistry* 33:518-523.

Nhu, D. D., T. Kido, R. Naganuma, N. Swano, K. Tawara, M. Nishijo, H. Nakagawa, N. N. Hung, and L. T. H. Thom. 2009. A GIS study of dioxin contamination in a Vietnamese region sprayed with herbicide. *Environmental Health and Preventive Medicine* 14:353-360.

Pavlov, D. S., A. V. Smurov, L. V. Il'yash, D. N. Matorin, N. A. Kluyev, S. V. Kotelevtsev, V. S. Rumak, and T. G. Smurova. 2004. Present-day state of coral reefs in Nha Trang Bay (Southern Vietnam) and possible reasons for the disturbance of habitats of scleractinian coral. *Russian Journal of Marine Biology* 30(1):43-50.

Persson, N. J., L. T. Cousins, J. Molvaer, D. Broman, and K. Naes. 2006. Modeling the long-term fate of polychlorinated dibenzo-p-dioxins and furans (PCDD/Fs) in the Grenland Fjords, Norway. *Science of the Total Environment* 369:188-202.

Piazza, R., M. Sprovieri, M. L. Feo, R. Zangrando, M. Vecchiato, L. G. Bellucci, S. Guiliani, M. Frignani, N. H. Cu, and E. Marsella. 2007. PCDD/F hydrocarbons and pesticides in sediments of the Tam Giang-Cau Hai Lagoon, Central Vietnam. *Journal of Marine Science and Technology (Vietnam)* 1:102-109.

Podoll, R. T., H. M. Jaber, et al. (1986). Tetrachlorodibenzodioxin—Rates of volatilization and photolysis in the environment. *Environmental Science & Technology* 20(5):490-492.

Quinh, H. T., L. C. Dai, and L. T. H. Thom. 1989. Effects of geographical conditions, soil movement and other variables on the distribution of 2,3,7,8-TCDD levels in adipose tissues from Vietnam—Preliminary observations. *Chemosphere* 18(1-6):967-974.

Ross, J., and M. Ginevan. 2007. Points for the committee to consider when evaluating the Stellman model. Presentation to the IOM Committee on Making the Best Use of the Agent Orange Exposure Reconstruction Model. May 1.

Sauter, J. J., H. Kammerbauer, L. Pambor, and B. Hock. 1987. Evidence for the accelerated micromorphological degradation of epistomatal waxes in Norway spruce by motor vehicle emissions. *European Journal of Forest Pathology* 17(7):444-448.

Schecter, A., B. D. Eitzer, and R. A. Hites. 1989a. Chlorinated dioxin and dibenzofuran levels in sediments collected from rivers in Vietnam, 1984-6. *Chemosphere* 18(1-6):831-834.

Schecter, A., H. Y. Tong, S. J. Monson, and M. L. Gross. 1989b. Levels of 2,3,7,8-TCDD in silt samples collected between 1985-86 from rivers in the north and south of Vietnam. *Chemosphere* 19(1-6):547-550.

Schuler, F., P. Schmid, and C. Schlatter. 1998. Photodegradation of polychlorinated dibenzo-p-dioxins and dibenzofurans in cuticular waxes of laurel cherry (*Prunus laurocerasus*). *Chemosphere* 36(1):21-34.

Sinkkonen, S., and J. Paasivirta. 2000. Degradation half-life times of PCDDs, PCDFs and PCBs for environmental fate modeling. *Chemosphere* 40(9-11):943-949.

Sommerfreund, J. K., N. Gandhi, M. L. Diamond, C. Mugnai, M. Frignani, G. Capodaglio, M. Gerino, L. G. Bellucci, and S. Giuliani. 2010. Contaminant fate and transport in the Venice Lagoon: Results from a multi-segment multimedia model. *Ecotoxicology and Environmental Safety* 73(3):222-230.

Stellman, S. D., and J. M. Stellman. 2004. Exposure opportunity models for Agent Orange, dioxin, and other military herbicides used in Vietnam, 1961-1971. *Journal of Exposure Analysis and Environmental Epidemiology* 14(4):354-362.

Stellman, J. M., S. D. Stellman, R. Christian, T. Weber, and C. Tomasallo. 2003. The extent and patterns of usage of Agent Orange and other herbicides in Vietnam. *Nature* 422(6933):681-687.

Su, Y., F. Wania, Y. D. Lei, T. Harner, and M. Shoeib. 2007. Temperature dependence of the air concentrations of polychlorinated biphenyls and polybrominated diphenyl ethers in a forest and a clearing. *Environmental Science & Technology* 41(13):4655-4661.

Teske, M. E., S. L. Bird, D. M. Esterly, T. B. Curbishley, S. L. Ray, and S. G. Perry. 2002. AgDRIFT (R): A model for estimating near-field spray drift from aerial applications. *Environmental Toxicology and Chemistry* 21(3):659-671.

Ton, T. C. 1996. *Vietnam soil*. Hanoi, Vietnam: Agricultural Publishing House.

Turunen, M., and S. Hattunen. 1991. Effects of simulated acid rain on the epicuticular wax of Scots pine needles under northerly conditions. *Canadian Journal of Botany* 69:412-419.

van Jaarlsveld, J. A., and M. A. A. Schutter. 1993. Modeling the long-range transport and deposition of dioxins; first results for NW Europe. *Chemosphere* 27:131-139.

Wania, F., and M. S. McLachlan. 2001. Estimating the influence of forests on the overall fate of semivolatile organic compounds using a multimedia fate model. *Environmental Science & Technology* 35(3):582-590.

Ward, C. T., and F. Matsumura. 1978. Fate of 2,3,7,8-tetrachlorodibenzo-p-dioxin (TCDD) in a model aquatic environment. *Archives of Environmental Contamination and Toxicology* 7:349-357.

Young, A. L. 1983. Long-term studies on the persistence and movement of TCDD in a natural ecosystem. *Environmental Science Research* 26:173-190.

Young, A. L. 2009. *The history, use, disposition and environmental fate of Agent Orange*. New York, NY: Springer.

Zhang, H. J., J. P. Chen, Y. W. Ni, Q. Zhang, and L. Zhao. 2009. Uptake by roots and translocation to shoots of polychlorinated dibenzo-p-dioxins and dibenzofurans in typical crop plants. *Chemosphere* 76(6):740-746.

5

EXPOSURE ROUTES AND MECHANISMS

This committee was tasked with comparing exposure among three military populations that served in Vietnam—troops on the ground, Brown Water Navy personnel, and Blue Water Navy personnel—to Agent Orange and its contaminant, 2,3,7,8-tetrachlorodibenzo-p-dioxin (TCDD). Several previous Institute of Medicine (IOM) committees refrained from attempting to make precise estimates of troop-level exposure, because of the lack of data on concentrations of herbicides and particularly of the contaminant TCDD in air, water, soil, and foodstuffs during the Vietnam War and because of a paucity of information on the location of troops in relation to the location of spraying (IOM, 1994, 2003, 2008). Those uncertainties are amplified for Navy personnel, on whom even less information is available.

Thus, the approach used by this committee was to evaluate possible pathways of exposure of each of the three populations (termed exposure opportunities) and to consider whether it is plausible that people in these groups could have been exposed via these pathways to Agent Orange–associated TCDD. The lack of environmental concentration data and the lack of sufficient data on ground troop and Navy personnel locations made it impossible to quantify exposure for either of these populations. Thus, any assessment of exposure must be qualitative, rather than quantitative. Assessments of exposure opportunities were supported by information on the fate and transport of TCDD (see Chapter 4) and the sparse documented information on potential pathways of exposure. The committee also considered anecdotal information (including presentations given at its meetings) from a variety of sources.

The committee considered the environmental fate and transport of Agent orange–associated TCDD from aerial and riverbank spraying in combination with activities of Navy personnel and ground troops, as described in Chapter 4, as its starting point for its assessment of exposure opportunity. In the most general terms, environmental distribution processes, physical transport and dispersal, and degradation processes generally predict a concentration gradient for environmental herbicide and TCDD, with greater attenuation at greater distances from the points of introduction (spraying), except for processes that result in increasing concentrations, such as bioconcentration and distillation of marine water to make potable water on blue-water ships. It is therefore generally reasonable to suppose that the greatest exposure opportunities would be related to proximity to herbicide use and to locations with higher herbicide and TCDD contamination and that personnel who are at a distance from these locations would have lower exposures. Applying that general expectation to the circumstances and populations of interest has been the major thrust of the committee's efforts to characterize exposure. Specifically, the committee used fate and transport considerations combined with professional judgment to produce estimates of potential exposure opportunities in the three populations.

A schematic of the movement of Agent Orange and TCDD from the point of application (from spraying of Agent Orange from aircraft, from trucks, or from boats) to marine waters and air was shown in Figure 4-1. Working from that schematic, the committee sought to identify the exposure routes likely to result in Agent Orange and Agent Orange–associated TCDD exposure opportunities in each of the military populations. It should be noted that there are Blue Water Navy personnel who qualify as Brown Water Navy personnel as a result of their ships' locations or activities but have not yet been so designated by the Department of Veterans Affairs (VA), although they may be in the future. The committee did not consider the possible reclassification of those Blue Water Navy sailors in its exposure evaluations.

PREVIOUS EXPOSURE MODELING EFFORTS

Given their inability to quantify exposure of US military personnel to Agent Orange–associated TCDD, several prior IOM committees identified various approaches to approximate it. The IOM report *The Utility of Proximity-Based Herbicide Exposure Assessment in Epidemiologic Studies of Vietnam Veterans* (IOM, 2008) defined the simplest approach to characterizing herbicide exposure as being "based on a veteran's presence or absence in Vietnam during the period of herbicide spraying." At the second, more complex level, "measures of exposure ... are based on information on the location, timing, and volume of herbicide spraying combined with information on the location in space and time of individuals or military units." The measure might be refined at the third level by "incorporation of more detailed data or models for the fate and transport of herbicides in the environment, such as spray drift models, estimates of the proportion of the sprayed herbicide that reached the ground, or consideration of secondary transport of the herbicides or the TCDD contaminant in the environment." The fourth and fifth levels, as defined by that committee, begin to assess exposure at the individual level and require exposure and pharmacokinetic data.

Exposure opportunity has been defined as the *potential* for exposure rather than as a quantitative determination of exposure (that is, relatable to dose) and is therefore only a crude estimate of dose (IOM, 2008). There are no environmental concentration data (for example, data on concentrations in soil and water) for the three populations of interest on which to base estimates of individual dose or exposure levels. Thus, the *potential* for exposure is the best—in fact, the only—available method for assessing and comparing exposure.

To assess Blue Water Navy exposure opportunity, the committee expanded on past IOM definitions of exposure opportunity (beyond proximity to sprayed areas defined by the Stellman model (Stellman et al., 2003) and beyond exposure opportunity immediately after herbicide application) to include exposure pathways relevant to Blue Water Navy personnel (for example, shipboard treated water and accidental contact from coastal spraying).

EXPOSURE PATHWAYS

In conducting an exposure assessment for a site with active contamination, the standard approach would be to collect samples of various media, such as soil and water, and analyze them for chemicals of interest. However, there is no longer the opportunity to collect such data for the environmental media in Vietnam because the contamination occurred so long ago and it is virtually impossible to extrapolate from back from current TCDD concentrations to concentrations that might have been present during the Vietnam War. Therefore, two alternative approaches were considered. The first was to quantify exposure of the three populations (on the basis of the sparse data available on ground troops and Navy personnel movements and estimates of possible herbicide exposure in light of fate and transport considerations) and then compare ranges of exposure. Previous IOM committees (IOM, 2003, 2008) conducted exhaustive searches for sufficient information with which to conduct this type of assessment in connection with ground troops and concluded that such data were not available. The present committee sought data on the Blue Water Navy and similarly concluded that the necessary data are unavailable. Thus, the committee acknowledged the impossibility of this approach.

For the second approach, the committee determined that any assessment of exposure must be qualitative rather than quantitative. Qualitative estimates should be informed by knowledge of the fate and transport of the chemicals of interest and by documented or anecdotal information on potential pathways of exposure. The committee initially considered all potential exposure pathways, except spraying or other application and handling of herbicides, and then determined which of the potential routes could be considered plausible.

In the sections below, the committee examines the environmental pathways that could result in exposure of ground troops, Brown Water Navy personnel, and Blue Water Navy personnel to Agent Orange–associated TCDD from two major herbicide sources: aerial spraying and riverbank spraying. The committee discusses plausible pathways of exposure to TCDD in each environmental medium (air, soil and plants, freshwater, freshwater sediment, fish and other foods, and marine waters); determines whether each pathway can plausibly lead to Agent Orange–associated TCDD exposure; and presents the evidence on which the determination was based. Note that in the following sections, exposure of ground troops and Brown Water Navy personnel is considered together; the committee found that there is insufficient information on personnel behaviors, environmental concentrations of TCDD, or other crucial aspects of exposure to draw distinctions between exposures for these two populations. Figure 5-1 presents the exposure pathways the committee found to be plausible for ground troops, and Brown Water Navy personnel, and Blue Water Navy personnel.

The committee recognized that in addition to possible differences in exposure potential among populations, there are differences among individuals. Even ground troops or Navy personnel with similar job descriptions would be expected to have experienced varied exposure because of differences in environmental concentrations, personal activities, and associated intake characteristics (such as exposure duration, food and water ingestion rates, inhalation rate, and body weight). The committee recognizes that there may be individuals in a

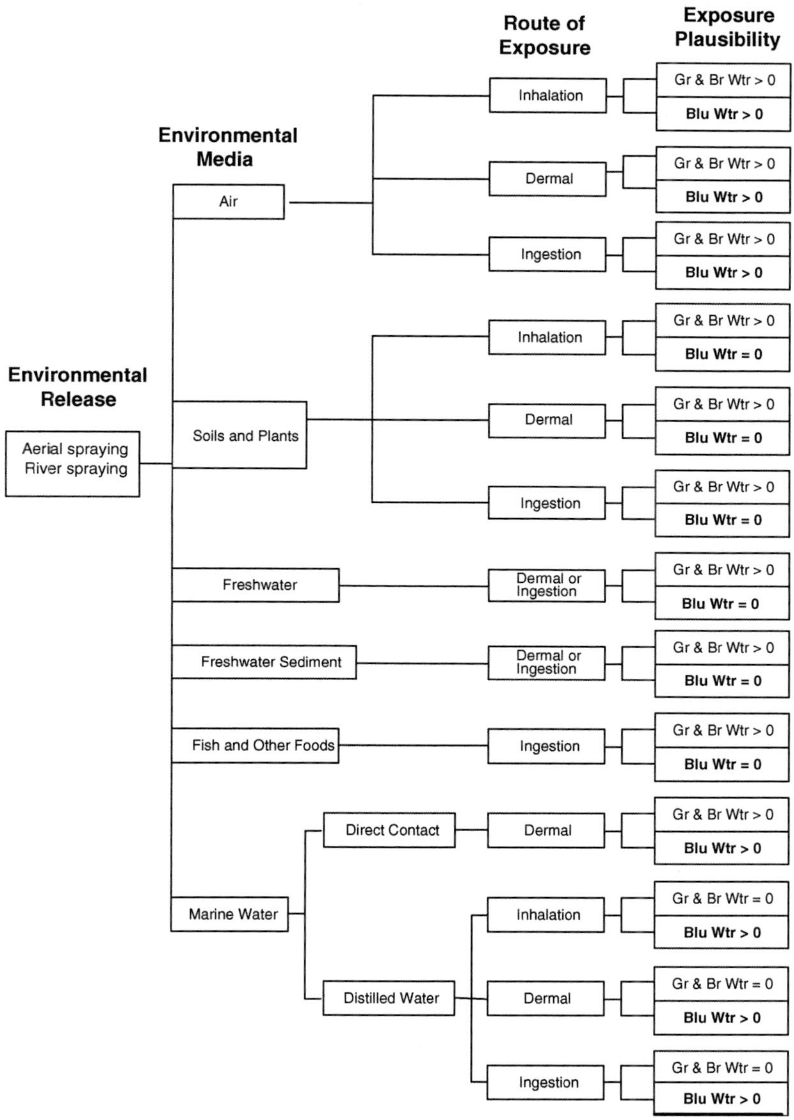

FIGURE 5-1 Exposure pathways for Agent Orange–associated TCDD.
NOTE: An exposure plausibility value of 0 indicates that this pathway is not considered to be plausible; a value of > 0 indicates that this pathway is considered to be plausible. Blu Wtr = Blue Water Navy personnel, Br Wtr = Brown Water Navy personnel, and Gr = ground troops.

given group whose experiences do not accord with the descriptions given in this report. It should be noted that ground troops and Brown Water Navy personnel included an unknown fraction of personnel who were remote from spraying operations and possibly had no opportunity for exposure. However, the VA noted that the definition of *ground troops who served in Vietnam* for the purposes of presumption of "service relatedness" was deliberately crafted to include persons who had little or no likelihood of exposure to guarantee that all cases of exposure (in the face of large uncertainties) were included. Thus, for the purposes of this report, if exposure was plausible for *any* fraction of a population, the committee assumed plausibility of exposure of the population as a whole. In addition, the committee recognizes that even a qualitative assessment of plausible exposure opportunity is fraught with uncertainty because of a lack of data, nonharmonious recollections of activities and locations of activities, and the heterogeneity of activities within each population.

Exposure to Agent Orange–Associated TCDD from Releases to Air

Herbicide and herbicide components exist in airborne form as aerosols from sprayed applications, as vapors of volatilizable herbicide components released from aerosols or from treated surfaces, and as aerosols from contaminated surfaces (soils, oil slicks, and marine surfaces) because of wind or mechanical action. Inhalation and dermal routes of exposure are considered, as well as ingestion, which is a plausible exposure route when aerosols and particles that enter the mouth are swallowed.

Inhalation

Ground troops and Brown Water Navy personnel

There is some information on ground troops and Brown Water Navy personnel on which to base conclusions regarding inhalation exposure plausibility (IOM, 2003, 2008). Although Young (2009) argues that ground troops were unlikely to be in or near areas of direct aerial spraying of herbicides, information on the distance between individual troops and the spray path is lacking. Given the possibility of spray drift of up to 7 km[1], the committee could not reject the possibility that some ground troops had inhalation exposure to herbicide spray drift. Stellman reported that during March 1969, 72 of 278 companies of Army combat battalions in III Corps Area were within 0.5 km of a spray path and had a potential for direct exposure to herbicide (IOM, 2008).

The General Accounting Office (now the Government Accountability Office) (GAO, 1979, cited in IOM, 2008, p. 49) found that 5,900 of 218,000 Marines who served in 1966–1969 were within 0.5 km of a spray path on the day of spraying and 17,400 were within 2.5 km; this suggests a potential for inhalation of spray drift. Brown Water Navy missions included some spraying of riverbank foliage, so in at least some instances Navy personnel were required to operate close to herbicide application. The committee was unable to ascertain how often that occurred or what proportion of Brown Water Navy personnel might have participated.

Therefore, although the extant information, based on modeling efforts, reveals variability in the extent of area over which troops and personnel may have plausibly inhaled Agent Orange–associated TCDD, common sense dictates that inhalation exposure of ground troops and Brown Water Navy personnel to Agent Orange spray drift or volatilized TCDD is plausible.[1]

Blue Water Navy personnel

The VA has determined that Blue Water Navy personnel do not have a presumption of exposure; this implies that their opportunity for herbicide exposure by aerial drift from spraying of herbicides in Vietnam was considered to be insignificant. The committee questioned that assumption. In the course of its deliberations, the committee was provided information indicating that many Blue Water Navy ships came relatively close to the Vietnamese shore, in some cases within 1 nautical mile of the coastline (RADM [retired] Joseph Carnevale, personal communication, June 9, 2010). Without data on the specific timing and location of each Operation Ranch Hand mission flown near the Vietnamese coastline and similar information on the timing and location of naval support missions, it is impossible to determine how many Blue Water Navy personnel might have been exposed to drift from aerial spraying and to what extent such exposure might have occurred near the coast. Maps of the Operation Ranch Hand missions, based on Herbicide Reporting System (HERBS) data, show that some flight paths were close to the South Vietnamese coast. In particular, there was heavy spraying in the III Corps Area near Saigon, including the mangrove swamps near the

[1]Estimates of extent of aerosol drift range from 2 to 7 km (Stellman et al., 2003; IOM, 2008) and up to 10 km (Department of the Army, 1971).

coast. It is plausible that drift from near-coastal spraying extended over estuarine and marine waters under some environmental conditions.

Without information to the contrary, the committee finds that it is plausible, although probably rare, that such exposure occurred. Therefore, the opportunity for Blue Water Navy personnel to have experienced inhalation exposure by this route cannot be entirely discounted but would have been limited to instances when vessels were operating close to (within a few kilometers of) shore in locations where and at times when spraying occurred.

Another source of potential inhalation exposure to Agent Orange was reported by Blue Water Navy veterans. The committee heard and read several anecdotal reports from Blue Water Navy personnel indicating that they had been sprayed from aircraft passing directly overhead. The committee is uncertain how to interpret those reports given the lack of specifics regarding the spraying incidents, such as where the ship was at the time of the incident (how far off the coast and where along the coast) and whether the spray was Agent Orange or another fluid, such as diesel fuel or malathion.

Stellman et al. (2003) identified about 40 cases of herbicide dumping in the HERBS files. The committee estimated that perhaps four of them were near the Vietnamese coast. The committee received one 1969 report indicating that one such dump occurred 10 km offshore in the South China Sea off Bac Lieu province, but information on the date, circumstances, and amount of the herbicide dump is not available (Susan Belanger, personal communication, November 28, 2010). That province is in the extreme south of Vietnam in an area that was heavily sprayed throughout the war. The committee considers inhalation exposure via aerial dumping of herbicides to have been very rare.

Ingestion

Ground troops and Brown Water Navy personnel

Ground troops and Brown Water Navy personnel might be expected to have some potential for ingestion of aerosols via inhalation followed by mucociliary transport and swallowing.

Blue Water Navy personnel

The committee could not rule out inhalation followed by mucociliary transport as a potential pathway of exposure of Blue Water Navy personnel who were aboard ships at sea.

Dermal

Ground troops and Brown Water Navy personnel

Direct deposition of herbicide spray onto any ground troops or Brown Water Navy personnel in the area of aerial spraying is possible and would be expected under conditions where there is substantial inhalation exposure opportunity. Young (2009) indicates that every effort was made to ensure that friendly ground troops were not in the vicinity of any of the Ranch Hand missions. Nevertheless, Stellman and Stellman (2004) indicate that some ground troops may have been in an area that could receive herbicide drift. Therefore, the committee concludes that some ground troops had the potential for direct dermal contact with herbicide-spray drift and could not rule out this pathway for Brown Water Navy personnel.

Blue Water Navy personnel

The committee's reasoning about dermal exposure of Blue Water Navy personnel from aerial drift follows the same line as for inhalation exposure. The lack of data on the extent of aerial drift and the different drift scenarios proposed by Stellman and Stellman (2004) and by Ross and Ginevan (2007) led the committee to conclude that, as with inhalation exposure, some level of dermal exposure might be possible for personnel aboard Blue Water Navy ships that were near shore (within the drift deposition area) during Ranch Hand missions. Similarly, dermal contact would be plausible if Blue Water Navy personnel were exposed to spray directly or from herbicide dumps. The committee recognizes that such instances may be rare, but they cannot be discounted entirely without further, labor-intensive efforts to coordinate Ranch Hand mission flight paths with Blue Water Navy ship locations.

Exposure to Agent Orange–Associated TCDD from Soils and Plants

Among the several factors that must be considered in assessing potential exposure to Agent Orange–associated TCDD via contact with soil or plants are penetration of the plant canopy to soil, adsorption of TCDD on plants and soil surfaces, dust concentrations in the atmosphere, and atmospheric degradation of volatilized Agent Orange–associated TCDD. Those fate and transport factors are discussed in Chapter 4.

Inhalation

Ground troops and Brown Water Navy personnel

Where Agent Orange has been used, adherence of TCDD to soil particles (dust) is likely. Dust may enter the atmosphere as a result of wind action across soil surfaces and mechanical actions, such as the movement of people or vehicles along unpaved surfaces. Ranch Hand missions and other herbicide-spraying missions often included clearing foliage from along roadways, and it is likely that ground troops and Brown Water Navy personnel inhaled dust if they entered a sprayed area before degradation of Agent Orange–associated TCDD occurred. Short-distance transport of contaminated dust can also occur, so even troops operating at some distance from the spray path might inhale the dust. Rain would act to remove dust particles from the air, and this would lead to the potential for additional contamination at some distance from the dust source as atmospheric washout.

Volatilization of TCDD from soil is possible, but the committee expects that only ground troops and Brown Water Navy personnel that were close to sprayed areas were likely to inhale Agent Orange–associated TCDD because of the potential for atmospheric dispersal and degradation of TCDD after volatilization from soil.

Inhalation exposure of ground troops and Brown Water Navy personnel could also have occurred as a result of the volatilization of Agent Orange–associated TCDD from plant surfaces (see Chapter 4) (Hornbuckle and Eisenreich, 1996; McLachlan et al., 2002), particularly as atmospheric temperatures rose through the day. Therefore, the committee determined that it is plausible that ground troops and Brown Water Navy personnel would have some opportunity for inhalation exposure to TCDD after aerial herbicide spraying and Agent Orange deposition on plant surfaces and soils.

Blue Water Navy personnel

Although volatilization of TCDD from plant surfaces and soil is possible and could result in the atmospheric transport of the chemical, the committee believes that—given the potential for photodegradation, dust washout in rain, and dispersal over long distances—it is unlikely that Blue Water Navy personnel would be exposed to Agent Orange–associated TCDD via this mechanism and route of exposure.

Ingestion

Ground troops and Brown Water Navy personnel

Ground troops might be expected to have some potential for ingestion of contaminated soils as a result of hand-to-mouth activity and consumption of foodstuffs and water contaminated with dust and dirt. That expectation is based on the likelihood of poor personal hygiene for many ground troops who lacked access to clean water and the likelihood that the same people passed through dusty areas where the soil had been contaminated by herbicide spraying. Another plausible mechanism for ingestion of Agent Orange–associated TCDD sorbed to dust is similar to that for ingestion of contaminated air discussed earlier, that is, movement of contaminated dust from the airways to the oropharynx. The committee could not rule out similar pathways of exposure of Brown Water Navy personnel.

Blue Water Navy personnel

The committee could not identify a plausible exposure pathway for ingestion of contaminated soil by Blue Water Navy personnel who were aboard ships at sea.

Dermal

Ground troops and Brown Water Navy personnel

Direct contact of ground troops and Brown Water Navy personnel with contaminated soil and sprayed foliage is possible. Dermal contact with contaminated soil is likely under circumstances similar to those of inhalation exposure to dust, that is, troops exposed to contaminated dust along roadways or other areas of exposed soil, to windblown dust, and possibly, for ground troops, from being obliged to lie on the soil for protection.

Ground troops in particular may come into contact with herbicide-sprayed vegetation, particularly if they enter a recently sprayed area. TCDD is known to adhere to the waxy surfaces of foliage (see Chapter 4). Ginevan et al. (2009) report that a conservative estimate of 20% of the amount of herbicide sprayed may be assumed to be available for transfer to human skin or clothing, but they also state that the bioavailability of TCDD on waxy leaf surfaces decreases rapidly, with a dissipation half-life of 1–3 days (Karch et al., 2004). Therefore, although it is difficult to determine how much TCDD is likely to transfer to ground troops entering a sprayed area within 3 days of spraying, such an exposure mechanism cannot be ruled out. A similar exposure scenario may be assumed for Brown Water Navy personnel brushing against foliage along riverbanks that have been sprayed.

Blue Water Navy personnel

Blue Water Navy personnel would not be expected to come into direct or indirect contact with contaminated Vietnamese soils or foliage while aboard ships at sea. Therefore, the committee concluded that there is no potential for exposure to Agent Orange–associated TCDD for Blue Water Navy personnel via this exposure pathway and route.

Exposure to Agent Orange–Associated TCDD from Fresh Water

Vietnam has numerous large and small rivers, streams, lakes, and bays that are used for transportation, fishing, and other activities. The committee was provided information that indicated that flight paths often included the spraying of surfaces of streams and rivers (Jeanne Stellman, Columbia University, presentation to the committee, September 20, 2010). In addition, Brown Water Navy personnel sprayed riverbanks (Zumwalt, 1993). Direct deposition of herbicide spray and, to a smaller extent, contaminated dust and atmospheric washout and water runoff are sources of herbicide contamination of surface waters (see Chapter 4). The committee did not consider inhalation exposure to Agent Orange–associated TCDD from contaminated surface waters to be an important route of exposure for any of the populations considered here.

Ingestion

Ground troops and Brown Water Navy personnel

The committee was unable to locate information on water sources or water treatment of Vietnamese surface (or ground) water to determine the potential for TCDD contamination of freshwater supplies either on US military bases or from local municipal water supplies. The committee was also unable to locate specific information about sources of potable water for ground troops and Brown Water Navy personnel. Westheider (2007) reported that water evaporators were used on some US military bases in Vietnam to produce potable water. Anecdotal information suggests that ground troops, particularly those who were in the field and away from firebases, would sometimes obtain their water from fast-running streams, rainwater, and shell holes in addition to carrying water canteens and rubber bladders (http://community.history.com/topic/

10831/t/Usable-water.html). Other information on water sources could not be identified. It is possible that some of the water sources had been sprayed with herbicide. Water treatment, if used, would probably be aimed at controlling pathogens and would not be expected to reduce TCDD contamination substantially other than by removal of settleable solids. Thus, exposure of the two populations to Agent Orange–associated TCDD via ingestion of freshwater is plausible.

Blue Water Navy personnel

Blue Water Navy ships generated their own potable water from marine water (discussed later) and therefore are not expected to have had the opportunity for exposure to potable water from Vietnamese freshwater sources. If a ship docked and took on potable water from Vietnam, crewmembers would have been eligible for a presumption of herbicide exposure only for the time the ship was docked (VA, 2008). Thus, exposure of this population to Agent Orange–associated TCDD via ingestion of freshwater was not considered to be plausible.

Dermal

Ground troops and Brown Water Navy personnel

Both ground troops and Brown Water Navy personnel had opportunities to come into direct contact with contaminated surface waters while wading through streams or along riverbanks or by entering the waters to swim or for other activities, such as boat repair. Thus, this route of exposure is plausible.

Blue Water Navy personnel

Blue Water Navy personnel are not expected to have had the opportunity for dermal contact with fresh surface waters unless their ship docked in Vietnam and took on freshwater. In that situation, crewmembers would be eligible for a presumption of herbicide exposure for the duration of the ship's docking.

Exposure to Agent Orange–Associated TCDD from Freshwater Sediment

The spraying of inland waters in Vietnam during the Operation Ranch Hand missions and reported riverbank spraying by Brown Water Navy personnel resulted in the contamination of surface waters. As described in Chapter 4, TCDD in water absorbs to organic material in the water and can be transported with the current or settle in sediment.

TCDD absorbed on soil particles could also enter the waterways via runoff from sprayed areas during rain or monsoons.

Ingestion

Ground troops and Brown Water Navy personnel

Ground troops and Brown Water Navy personnel might be expected to have some potential for ingestion of contaminated sediments as a result of consumption of water that contained sediments. Hand-to-mouth activity may also result in ingestion where hygiene is poor.

Blue Water Navy personnel

Blue Water Navy personnel are not expected to have had opportunities for exposure to freshwater sediments in the inland waters of Vietnam.

Dermal

Ground troops and Brown Water Navy personnel

As in the case of exposure to contaminated surface waters, ground troops and Brown Water Navy personnel may have had the opportunity for direct contact with contaminated sediments when walking along riverbanks, wading across streams, or engaged in other activities in inland waters, such as swimming. Because sediments can be transported for some distance in water with a strong current, it is possible that military personnel were exposed to TCDD-contaminated sediments even when they were not near sprayed areas.

Blue Water Navy personnel

Blue Water Navy personnel are not expected to have had opportunities for exposure to freshwater sediments in the inland waters of Vietnam.

Exposure to Agent Orange–Associated TCDD from Fish and Other Foods

Most human exposure to TCDD via food comes from the consumption of contaminated animal products, such as meat, fish, and dairy. Animals may eat contaminated forage, such as grasses, and bioaccumulate TCDD in their fatty tissues (IOM, 2003). Although TCDD is poorly translocated in plants (Zhang et al., 2009) and TCDD that adheres to plant surfaces typically does not move to other plant parts, animals and humans may consume TCDD in contaminated soil particles that adhere to the plants if they are not thoroughly cleaned before consumption. Fish are also likely to bioaccumulate TCDD from water via ingestion of contaminated organic matter (Rifkin and Lakind, 1991; Chiao et al., 1994).

Ingestion

Ground troops and Brown Water Navy personnel

The opportunity for exposure to TCDD-contaminated food varied considerably among military personnel stationed in Vietnam. Reports indicate that much of the food of US military personnel stationed on larger bases was obtained from the United States as rations. Westheider (2007) states that "at base camps, soldiers ate a variety of foods, from steak and potatoes washed down with beer to Vietnamese dishes in local eateries." Other military personnel, particularly Army soldiers and Marines, were issued or otherwise had available C rations. US Air Force and Navy personnel most often had access to dining facilities that served a greater variety of food, including A rations.

Long Range Reconnaissance Patrol rations contained freeze-dried foods (http://wiki.answers.com/Q/Food_available_at_the_vietnam_war). Food in the field included a variety of dehydrated and canned meals or fish, rice, and food obtained from the vicinity. Field kitchens would serve B rations, 1-gal cans of food prepared by Army cooks in the field (Westheider, 2007).

US Navy riverine forces would have consumed C rations while patrolling the rivers in their boats (http://www.pbs.org/wgbh/amex/vietnam/trenches/weapons.html).

TCDD concentrations in the food obtained from the United States is expected to be the same as would be experienced by the majority of the US population. The committee was unable to obtain any measurements of the TCDD content of local Vietnamese foods during the war. Because local foods were consumed and some local foods may have been derived from crops grown in areas that had been sprayed with herbicides or derived from animals that had grazed on herbicide-sprayed crops, the committee could not rule out consumption of food as a pathway for exposure of the two populations to Agent Orange–associated TCDD.

Blue Water Navy personnel

Blue Water Navy ships did not take on rations of Vietnamese food but relied on rations of US food or food from other locations, such as

Subic Bay, Philippines. Thus, they would not have had the opportunity for Agent Orange–associated TCDD exposure via ingestion of contaminated foods. The committee was informed that the Blue Water Navy ships rarely or never obtained food from Vietnam. That is consistent with the information received by the committee during its public session on the *USS Midway* regarding the operation of the larger ships, such as aircraft carriers, but the committee was unable to determine whether there might have been exceptions among smaller ships that operated in coastal marine waters. Blue Water Navy personnel on ships that docked in Vietnam to take on food, including Vietnamese food, would meet the criteria for a presumption of herbicide exposure if they stated they went ashore while the ship was docked.

The committee heard conflicting reports on whether fishing from Blue Water Navy ships occurred. Some indicated that there was occasional fishing and consumption of the fish caught. Others indicated that fishing from their ships was nonexistent. In the absence of data beyond the testimony on fishing and fish-consumption practices, such an exposure mechanism cannot be ruled out, although the amount of TCDD consumed by eating contaminated marine fish is likely to be very small.

Exposure to Agent Orange–Associated TCDD from Marine Water

The concentrations of TCDD in the marine waters surrounding Vietnam during the war have been the subject of much debate and considerable speculation. No contemporaneous measurements of TCDD in marine waters or sediments were identified by the committee. As discussed in Chapter 4 and the Appendix, TCDD tends to adsorb on organic matter in water; thus, freshwater that contains suspended organic matter and enters marine systems from areas that were treated with herbicides is likely to have contained Agent Orange–associated TCDD. Contamination of marine waters by direct application or discharge of Agent Orange is also a possible scenario. Records of spraying of Agent Orange over marine waters as part of Operation Ranch Hand have not been identified. The committee did not examine all the HERBS files to determine whether any of the Ranch Hand missions sprayed herbicides intentionally or accidentally over marine waters. However, some of the flight paths, such as those over the Rung Sat area, appear to have extended to coastal waters, albeit for only short distances. There are rare reports of Ranch Hand aircraft dumping herbicide over coastal waters (10 km offshore), as noted earlier. Moreover, the committee heard and read several anecdotal reports of aircraft spraying over marine waters. The committee was unable to locate any confirmed reports of Agent Orange spraying over marine waters.

The committee considered that some direct contact of all the military populations stationed in and around South Vietnam with TCDD-contaminated marine water was possible. The only plausible route of exposure to TCDD in marine waters is dermal contact. On the basis of the best professional judgment, the committee did not consider exposure via contaminated marine water by ingestion or inhalation as plausible. The exception is the use of distilled marine water as potable water on Blue Water Navy ships; this is discussed separately below.

Dermal Contact

Ground troops and Brown Water Navy personnel

There are numerous pictures of American troops in marine waters—for example, at China Beach—during the war (for example, http://www.wardogs.com/vcbcbl.html). Those personnel may have been exposed to Agent Orange–associated TCDD by swimming or wading in contaminated waters. Although no specific information on Brown Water Navy personnel was available, they might have been exposed to Agent Orange–associated TCDD in marine waters if they were operating near the mouth of a river that was contaminated or if their ship moved from brown water to blue water and they were in contact with the water.

Blue Water Navy personnel

The committee was told that personnel on larger ships operating off the coast did not engage in marine swimming, but it was within the discretion of the commanding officer of each ship to permit it. The committee heard anecdotal reports of occasional swim calls on some smaller Blue Water Navy ships. The committee was told that such calls were infrequent because of the dangers associated with sharks and sea snakes in the South China Sea. Therefore, although the committee found it plausible that Blue Water Navy personnel may have had occasional direct dermal contact with contaminated marine waters from swimming or spray (during heavy seas), such contact was expected to be infrequent and of short duration.

Distilled Potable Water

Blue Water Navy personnel

Large Blue Water Navy ships—such as aircraft carriers, cruisers, and destroyers—generated their own potable-water supply for use in ships' boilers and secondarily for crew uses, such as drinking, food preparation, bathing, and cleaning. Potable water is produced by distillation of marine water. Although the marine water passed through a sieve to remove large debris such as seaweed, the water was not further filtered or treated before it entered the ship's distillation plant. The use of shipboard distillation plants is discussed in more detail in the Appendix. As a matter of policy, production of potable water from polluted marine waters, such as estuaries and harbors or when ships are traveling in close formation, was avoided (NAVMED P-5010-6) (Department of the Navy, 1990). Section 2.4.2, "Polluted Water" of the *Naval Ships' Technical Manual*, states that

> unless determined otherwise, water in harbors, rivers, inlets, bays, landlocked waters, and the open sea within 12 miles of the entrance to these waterways, shall be considered to be polluted.... The desalting of polluted harbor water or seawater for human consumption shall be avoided except in emergencies.

The committee was unable to determine whether this regulation was in effect during the Vietnam War but was told by several retired naval officers that it was the practice at that time, although exceptions did occur. The committee received information from several Blue Water Navy veterans that firing lines for US ships could be as close to the Vietnamese coastline as 1–2 nautical miles. Although ships did not stay on the firing line for long periods, it is possible that they sometimes took up water for distillation while relatively close to the coastline.

The issue of distillation of marine water is important because of the finding by the committee that prepared the 2008 *Veterans and Agent Orange* update (IOM, 2008) that Blue Water Navy veterans could have been exposed to TCDD via contaminated potable water. As noted in that report and discussed in the Appendix to the present report, the Australian Department of Veterans Affairs determined that Royal Australian Navy personnel who served offshore were exposed to TCDD from herbicide spraying in Vietnam because the distillation systems onboard the ships were thought to be able to increase the concentration of TCDD in potable water during the evaporative process compared with the TCDD concentration in the source water (Muller et al., 2001). In the Appendix, a theoretical model is applied to a batch distillation model by using physical constants of TCDD to corroborate the findings of the experimental Australian study that found substantial codistillation of contaminants during production of potable water with a batch distillation unit. The findings of the theoretical model agreed with the findings of the Australian study that codistillation was probable during distillation of contaminated water. Therefore, high contaminant concentrations in source water could be magnified during the distillation process. If Agent Orange–associated TCDD was present in the marine water, potable water was a plausible route of exposure.

As presented in Chapter 4, the committee found that Agent Orange–associated TCDD could, under some circumstances, contaminate marine waters off the coast of South Vietnam. Blue Water Navy ships may have distilled those marine waters, so TCDD contamination of potable water aboard those ships was possible. Use of potable water containing Agent Orange–associated TCDD could result in inhalation exposure to TCDDs in water vapor during showering or other uses of hot water, such as cooking, and could result in volatilization of TCDD from the water during other uses, such as cleaning. Use of the water for showering and cleaning would also result in dermal exposure to TCDDs. Finally, the use of the potable water for drinking itself and for food preparation could lead to ingestion of TCDD. Questions about the engineering systems used to produce potable water on Blue Water Navy ships and their effect on concentrations or enrichment of Agent Orange–associated TCDD increase the uncertainty in the importance of this exposure route.

CONCLUSIONS

The committee identified several plausible exposure pathways and routes of exposure to Agent Orange–associated TCDD in the three populations, including Blue Water Navy personnel (see Figure 5-1). Plausible pathways and routes of exposure of Blue Water Navy personnel to Agent Orange–associated TCDD include inhalation and dermal contact with aerosols from spraying operations that occurred at or near the coast when Blue Water Navy ships were nearby, contact with marine water, and uses of distilled water prepared from marine water.

The committee cannot provide quantitative estimates of exposure by any of the exposure pathways described above because of lack of data on environmental concentrations of TCDD and activity patterns of military personnel. At best, the committee can judge whether specific routes of exposure are plausible.

REFERENCES

Chiao, F. F., R. C. Currie, and T. E. McKone. 1994. Intermedia transfer factors for contaminants found at hazardous waste sites: 2,3,7,8-tetrachlorodibenzo-p-dioxin (TCDD). Davis, CA: University of California, Davis.

Department of the Army. 1971. *Field manual: Tactical employment of herbicides*. Washington, DC: Headquarters. December.

Department of the Navy. 1990. Chapter 533, Potable Water Systems. *Navy ships' technical manual*. NAVMED P-5010-6. Washington, DC: Naval Sea Systems Command.

Ginevan, M. E., J. H. Ross, and D. K. Watkins. 2009. Assessing exposure to allied ground troops in the Vietnam War: A comparison of AgDRIFT and Exposure Opportunity Index models. *Journal of Exposure Science and Environmental Epidemiology* 19(2):187-200.

Hornbuckle, K. C., and S. J. Eisenreich. 1996. Dynamics of gaseous semivolatile organic compounds in a terrestrial ecosystem—Effects of diurnal and seasonal climate variations. *Atmospheric Environment* 30:3935-3945.

IOM (Institute of Medicine). 1994. *Veterans and Agent Orange: Health effects of herbicides used in Vietnam.* Washington, DC: National Academy Press.

IOM. 2003. *Characterizing exposure of veterans to Agent Orange and other herbicides used in Vietnam.* Washington, DC: The National Academies Press.

IOM. 2008. *The utility of proximity-based herbicide exposure assessment in epidemiologic studies of Vietnam veterans*. Washington, DC: The National Academies Press.

Karch, N. J., D. K. Watkins, A. L. Young, and M. E. Ginevan. 2004. Environmental fate of TCDD and Agent Orange and bioavailability to troops in Vietnam. *Organohalogen Compounds* 66.

McLachlan, M. S., G. Czub, and F. Wania. 2002. The influence of vertical sorbed phase transport on the fate of organic chemicals in surface soils. *Environmental Science & Technology* 36(22):4860-4867.

Muller, J. F., C. Gaus, K. Bundred, V. Alberts, M. R. Moore, and K. Horsley. 2002. *Examination of the potential exposure of Royal Australian Navy (RAN) personnel to polychlorinated dibenzodioxins and polychlorinated dibenzofurans via drinking water. A report to: The Department of Veteran Affairs, Australia.* Brisbane, Australia: National Research Centre for Environmental Toxicology.

Rifkin, E., and J. Lakind. 1991. Dioxin bioaccumulation: Key to a sound risk assessment methodology. *Journal of Toxicology and Environmental Health* 33(1):103-112.

Ross, J., and M. Ginevan. 2007. Points for the committee to consider when evaluating the Stellman model. Presentation to the IOM Committee on Making the Best Use of the Agent Orange Exposure Reconstruction Model. May 1.

Stellman, S. D., and J. M. Stellman. 2004. Exposure opportunity models for Agent Orange, dioxin, and other military herbicides used in Vietnam, 1961-1971. *Journal of Exposure Analysis and Environmental Epidemiology* 14(4):354-362.

Stellman, J. M., S. D. Stellman, R. Christian, T. Weber, and C. Tomasallo. 2003. The extent and patterns of usage of Agent Orange and other herbicides in Vietnam. *Nature* 422(6933):681-687.

VA (Department of Veterans Affairs). 2008. Further definition of Vietnam "Blue Water" versus "Brown Water" service for the purpose of determining Agent Orange exposure. *Compensation & Pension Service Bulletin* p. 2-3. December.

Westheider, J. E. 2007. *The Vietnam War.* Westport, CT: Greenwood Press.

Young, A. L. 2009. *The history, use, disposition and environmental fate of Agent Orange.* New York, NY: Springer.

Zhang, H., J. Chen, Y. Ni, Q. Zhang, and L Zhao. 2009. Uptake by roots and translocation to shoots of polychlorinated dibenzo-p-dioxins and dibenzofurans in typical crop plants. *Chemosphere* 76(6):740-746.

Zumwalt, E. R. 1993. *Letter to the Institute of Medicine Committee to Review the Health Effects in Vietnam Veterans of Exposure to Herbicides regarding draft version of the IOM chapter on the U.S. military and the herbicide program in Vietnam*, May 20, 1993.

6

LONG-TERM ADVERSE HEALTH EFFECTS

The long-term health effects associated with exposure to dioxins have been studied in a variety of populations, including Vietnam veterans and residents of Seveso, Italy, the site of an accidental release of dioxin. The biennial Institute of Medicine (IOM) *Veterans and Agent Orange* (*VAO*) reports have reviewed epidemiologic studies of Vietnam veterans, occupational studies, and population studies in an effort to determine whether Vietnam veterans are at increased risk for health effects from exposure to Agent Orange and its contaminant 2,3,7,8-tetrachlorodibenzo-p-dioxin (also referred to as TCDD) during the Vietnam War. The literature is voluminous, and the *VAO* reports have been updated through 2008. A few of the studies include veterans who served in the Blue Water Navy in Vietnam, but most of the studies do not distinguish Navy veterans, let alone Blue Water Navy veterans, from other Vietnam-veteran populations.

In compliance with the congressional legislation that mandated the biennial reports, the VAO committees have examined the available evidence of a positive association between Agent Orange and health outcomes from epidemiologic studies in which chance, bias, and confounding can be ruled out with reasonable confidence. The committees have assigned the association to the following categories: sufficient evidence of association, limited or suggestive evidence of association, inadequate or insufficient evidence to determine association, and limited or suggestive evidence of no association (see Table 6-1). The reviews of the literature can be found in the eight *VAO* reports and are not repeated here; Table 6-1 summarizes these findings. The findings by the VAO committees regarding health effects for which there is sufficient evidence of an association are not identical to the list of diseases that the Department of Veterans Affairs (VA) recognizes as

TABLE 6-1 Summary of Seventh Biennial Update of Findings of Occupational, Environmental, and Veteran Studies Regarding Associations Between Exposure to Herbicides and Specific Health Outcomes[a]

Sufficient Evidence of an Association

Epidemiologic evidence is sufficient to conclude that there is a positive association. That is, a positive association has been observed between exposure to herbicides and the outcome in studies in which chance, bias, and confounding could be ruled out with reasonable confidence.[b] For example, if several small studies that are free of bias and confounding show an association that is consistent in magnitude and direction, there could be sufficient evidence of an association. There is sufficient evidence of an association between exposure to the chemicals of interest and the following health outcomes:

- Soft-tissue sarcoma (including heart), *1994 (year of IOM finding), 1990 (year of VA service-connection decision)*
- Non-Hodgkin's lymphoma, *1994, 1990*
- Chronic lymphocytic leukemia (including hairy-cell leukemia and other chronic B-cell leukemias) (category clarification since *Update 2006*), *2003, 2004*
- Hodgkin's disease, *1994, 1995*
- Chloracne, *1994, 1985*

Limited or Suggestive Evidence of an Association

Epidemiologic evidence suggests an association between exposure to herbicides and the outcome, but a firm conclusion is limited because chance, bias, and confounding could not be ruled out with confidence. For example, a well-conducted study that had strong findings in accord with less compelling results from studies of populations with similar exposures could constitute such evidence. There is limited or suggestive evidence of an association between exposure to the chemicals of interest and the following health outcomes:

- Laryngeal cancer, *1994, 1995*
- Cancer of the lung, bronchus, or trachea, *1994, 1995*
- Prostatic cancer, *1994, 1997*
- Multiple myeloma, *1994, 1995*
- AL amyloidosis, *2007, 2009*
- Early-onset transient peripheral neuropathy, *1996, 1997*
- Parkinson's disease (category change from *Update 2006*), *2009, 2009*
- Porphyria cutanea tarda, *1994*; *sufficient, 1996*; changed to *limited or suggestive, 1995*

TABLE 6-1 Summary of Seventh Biennial Update of Findings of Occupational, Environmental, and Veteran Studies Regarding Associations Between Exposure to Herbicides and Specific Health Outcomes[a]

- Hypertension *2007*, not VA service connected
- Ischemic heart disease (category change from *Update 2006*), *2009*, *2009*
- Type 2 diabetes (mellitus), *2000*, *2001*
- Spina bifida in offspring of exposed people, *1996*, *1996*

Inadequate or Insufficient Evidence to Determine an Association

The available epidemiologic studies are of insufficient quality, consistency, or statistical power to permit a conclusion regarding the presence or absence of an association. For example, studies fail to control for confounding, have inadequate exposure assessment, or fail to address latency. There is inadequate or insufficient evidence to determine an association between exposure to the chemicals of interest and the following health outcomes that were explicitly reviewed:

- Cancers of the oral cavity (including lips and tongue), pharynx (including tonsils), or nasal cavity (including ears and sinuses)
- Cancers of the pleura, mediastinum, and other unspecified sites in the respiratory system and intrathoracic organs
- Esophageal cancer
- Stomach cancer
- Colorectal cancer (including small intestine and anus)
- Hepatobiliary cancers (liver, gallbladder, and the bile ducts)
- Pancreatic cancer
- Bone and joint cancer
- Melanoma
- Nonmelanoma skin cancer (basal-cell and squamous-cell)
- Breast cancer
- Cancers of the reproductive organs (cervix, uterus, ovary, testis, and penis; excluding prostate)
- Urinary bladder cancer
- Renal cancer (kidney and renal pelvis)
- Cancers of brain and nervous system (including eye)
- Endocrine cancers (thyroid, thymus, and other endocrine organs)
- Leukemia (other than all chronic B-cell leukemias, such as chronic lymphocytic leukemia and hairy-cell leukemia)
- Cancers at other and unspecified sites
- Infertility

TABLE 6-1 Summary of Seventh Biennial Update of Findings of Occupational, Environmental, and Veteran Studies Regarding Associations Between Exposure to Herbicides and Specific Health Outcomes[a]

- Spontaneous abortion (other than after paternal exposure to TCDD, which appears not to be associated)
- Neonatal or infant death and stillbirth in offspring of exposed people
- Low birth weight in offspring of exposed people
- Birth defects (other than spina bifida) in offspring of exposed people
- Childhood cancer (including acute myelogenous leukemia) in offspring of exposed people
- Neurobehavioral disorders (cognitive and neuropsychiatric)
- Neurodegenerative diseases, excluding Parkinson's disease
- Chronic peripheral nervous system disorders
- Respiratory disorders (wheeze or asthma, chronic obstructive pulmonary disease, and farmer's lung)
- Gastrointestinal, metabolic, and digestive disorders (changes in hepatic enzymes, lipid abnormalities, and ulcers)
- Immune system disorders (immune suppression, allergy, and autoimmunity)
- Circulatory disorders (other than hypertension and ischemic heart disease)
- Endometriosis
- Effects on thyroid homeostatis

The VAO committees used a classification that spans the full array of cancers. However, reviews for nonmalignant conditions were conducted only if they were found to have been the subjects of epidemiologic investigation or at the request of the VA. By default, any health outcome on which no epidemiologic information has been found falls into this category.

TABLE 6-1 Summary of Seventh Biennial Update Findings of Occupational, Environmental, and Veteran Studies Regarding Associations Between Exposure to Herbicides and Specific Health Outcomes[a]

Limited or Suggestive Evidence of *No* Association

Several adequate studies, which cover the full range of human exposure, are consistent in not showing a positive association between any magnitude of exposure to the herbicides of interest and the outcome. A conclusion of "no association" is inevitably limited to the conditions, exposures, and length of observation covered by the available studies. *In addition, the possibility of a very small increase in risk at the exposure studied can never be excluded.* There is limited or suggestive evidence of *no* association between exposure to the herbicides of interest and the following health outcomes:

- Spontaneous abortion after paternal exposure to TCDD, *2002*

[a]Herbicides indicates the following chemicals of interest: 2,4-dichlorophenoxyacetic acid (2,4-D), 2,4,5-trichlorophenoxyacetic acid (2,4,5-T) and its contaminant 2,3,7,8-tetrachlorodibenzo-p-dioxin (TCDD), cacodylic acid, and picloram. The evidence regarding association was drawn from occupational, environmental, and veteran studies in which people were exposed to the herbicides used in Vietnam, to their components, or to their contaminant.
[b]Evidence of an association is strengthened by experimental data that support biologic plausibility, but its absence would not detract from the epidemiologic evidence.
SOURCE: Adapted from IOM (2009) and annotated to indicate the year of IOM finding and year of VA service connection.

linked to herbicide exposure in Vietnam and for which compensation is provided. Decisions regarding compensation are made by the VA, which takes both the *VAO* reports and other factors into consideration. For example, the VA recognizes non-Hodgkin's lymphoma (NHL) as a service-related condition in Vietnam veterans, including Blue Water Navy veterans, but does not link it to Agent Orange exposure, although the VA website on these diseases does (http://www.publichealth.va.gov/exposures/diseases.asp).

In addition to reviewing previous *VAO* reports, the present committee heard from a number of veterans and is aware that many veterans attribute their illnesses to exposure to Agent Orange in Vietnam. The committee valued these accounts for descriptive purposes but did not have a way to use that information effectively in its study. Without an appropriate control population and representative sample of Blue Water Navy veterans, the committee was unable to determine if these veterans' diseases could be attributed to Agent Orange–associated TCDD exposure. This committee was asked to assess the potential long-term health effects of exposure to herbicides in Blue Water Navy Vietnam veterans as a population distinct from other Vietnam veterans, as the VA compensates veterans based on the presumption of exposure for specific groups such as ground troops. To do that, the committee examined only peer-reviewed epidemiologic studies that identified Blue Water Navy Vietnam veterans as a separate population. Since individual exposure to TCDD could not be estimated (see Chapter 5), the committee could not determine any dose-response relationships for health effects experienced by Blue Water Navy veterans. The committee attempted to determine whether adverse health outcomes among Blue Water Navy personnel were consistent with those associated with TCDD exposure in other Vietnam veterans and if their health effects occurred more or less frequently than those seen in other Vietnam veterans previously identified as exposed to TCDD.

VIETNAM VETERAN STUDIES

Although the subjects of many epidemiologic studies of Vietnam veterans include Navy veterans, the committee found only a few studies that examined Vietnam Navy personnel specifically as a study population (the methods of the literature search are described in Chapter 1). Whether the Navy population in question was Blue Water Navy, was Brown Water Navy, or served on land in Vietnam or elsewhere was rarely indicated. The studies are presented below alphabetically by author.

Australian's Vietnam Veteran Mortality and Cancer-Incidence Studies

In 2005, the Australian Institute of Health and Welfare of the Department of Veterans' Affairs released the results of a series of reports investigating mortality and cancer incidence in Australian veterans. Two of the reports focused specifically on the health of Vietnam veterans (Wilson et al., 2005a,b). The 59,179 male Australian veterans who served in Vietnam between 1962–1973, were retrospectively followed to assess mortality and cancer outcomes. Data were provided by the Australian Department of Veterans' Affairs Nominal Roll of Vietnam Veterans. Cancers diagnosed from 1982 through 2000 and deaths occurring after service in Vietnam through 2001 were compared with those in the general population of Australian men. Mortality and incidence were standardized for age and calendar year.

The 57,864 veterans included in the analysis had 4,590 cancers. Overall, the incidence of all cancers in the entire Australian Vietnam veteran population was increased by 13–15% compared to the general male population; the highest rates were found in the 12,935 Navy veterans, in whom the overall incidence of cancer (1,073 cancers) was 22–26% higher than in the control population. With regard to specific cancers, in the Navy veteran population, the incidences of the following cancers were found to be statistically significantly higher: lung cancer[1] (relative risk [RR] 1.4, 95% CI 1.2–1.7), head and neck cancers (RR 1.6, 95% CI 1.1–2.0), melanoma (RR 1.4, 95% CI 1.2–1.6), and colon cancer (RR 1.3, 95% CI 1.0–1.5). The incidences of leukemia,[1] brain cancer, laryngeal cancer,[1] Hodgkin's disease,[1] prostatic cancer,[1] and esophageal cancer were also higher but the difference was not statistically significant. The incidence of one cancer linked to Agent Orange exposure, NHL,[1] was found to be lower than that in the control population (RR 0.8, 95% CI 0.5–1.0) (Wilson et al., 2005a).

A ship-by-ship analysis found no significant differences in cancer rates between specific ships or types of ships or compared with a control ship, the HMAS *Melbourne,* which was in the Vietnam theater but never served near the coast. Time spent on ships in Vietnamese waters also did not correlate with a difference in cancer incidence. The study authors concluded that "this study did not, therefore, provide any evidence to support the hypothesis that the increased cancer rates seen among Navy personnel could be attributable to exposure to contaminated water" (Wilson et al., 2005c). The analysis of standardized incidence ratios (SIRs) included only the larger ships due to power considerations.

The Australian Vietnam veterans had an overall mortality that was 6% lower (on the basis of 6,166 deaths) than that in the general male population, but the disparity in rates was present for only the first 20

---

[1]The IOM *VAO* reports have found sufficient or limited/suggestive evidence of association between this condition and exposure to herbicides.

years after the war and was comparable in the two populations as of 2001. Mortality in Navy veterans (1,435 deaths) was also comparable with that in the general population except for cancer deaths—overall mortality from cancer was 19% higher. The greatest differences were seen in lung cancer (RR 1.4, 95% CI 1.2–1.6), melanoma (RR 1.6, 95% CI 1.0–2.1), and mesothelioma (RR 2.53, 95% CI 1.11–4.94). Mortality from NHL was 48% lower (RR 0.5, 95% CI 0.3–0.9). Several other causes of mortality were significantly lower, including, diabetes, mental and behavioral disorders, and respiratory disorders. For lung cancer, oral cancer, head and neck cancer, and prostatic cancer, both incidence and mortality were higher; for NHL, they were lower (Wilson et al., 2005b).

The studied cohort of Australian Vietnam veterans is large and included a long follow-up period; the cohort is fairly homogeneous (male, mostly white, and able to meet military physical, medical, and educational standards), and only 2.5% were lost to follow-up. However, some degree of error is expected with the probabilistic matching used to ascertain outcomes from cancer and death registries linked to the Nominal Roll of Vietnam Veterans (rather than exact matching between veteran data and registries), possibly causing cancer and death outcomes to have been missed or wrongly assigned to veterans. Individual data pertaining to specific exposures in the military or before or after active duty were not available, so the results described represent an overall average exposure scenario for veterans. The authors also note the potential for a healthy-warrior effect inasmuch as the military actively screens personnel for health problems, so they are healthier than the general population, and risk estimates are lower. The healthy-worker effect is not seen in Navy veterans as the all-cause mortality rate is similar to that of the general population. Finally, the Australian analyses did not control for confounding variables, such as smoking.

Bullman et al.

This case–control study compared the incidence of testicular cancer in Vietnam veterans with different probable exposures to Agent Orange (Bullman et al., 1994). Ninety-seven veteran cases were identified from voluntary VA Agent Orange Registry medical examinations in 1982–1991 and matched with 311 controls: 67 Army cases with 218 controls, 10 Air Force cases with 22 controls, eight Marines cases with 56 controls, and 12 Navy cases with 15 controls. Controls were identified from the same registry but had no clinical diagnosis on record. In the absence of specific information about exposure levels, surrogate measures of Agent Orange exposure were used, including service branch, type of duty, corps area, and location of ground troops. The analysis did not adjust for confounding, because there were no effects of race and age after stratification.

The only veteran exposure group with a higher incidence of testicular cancer was the Navy group (crude odds ratio [OR] 2.60, 95% CI 1.08–6.24). None of the Navy veterans who had testicular cancer served in the Brown Water Navy, and only one of the 15 Navy controls did so. The authors assumed that the Navy exposure group had lower Agent Orange exposure than ground troops and concluded that "the study results are not consistent with the hypothesis that Agent Orange may be a risk factor for testicular cancer among Vietnam veterans."

Bullman and colleagues note several limitations and biases potentially affecting their results. Interpretation of those results should consider the lack of adjustment for confounders and other exposures (race, exposure to fuels, etc.) and the potentially poor ability of surrogate exposure measures to represent actual exposure. Exposure misclassification is an important limitation in that "unexposed" troops may have been exposed by being in areas after Agent Orange spraying even if they did not work directly with the chemicals. Thus service branch may be a poor proxy for exposure. Likewise, military records are reportedly a poor source of information for estimating Agent Orange exposure.

Centers for Disease Control and Prevention Selected Cancers Study

For evaluating cancer risks in Blue Water Navy Vietnam veterans, the most informative study was the Selected Cancers Study conducted by the Centers for Disease Control and Prevention (CDC) (1990a,b,c). Population-based case–control studies of American men born in 1929–1953 were designed to determine the incidence of rare cancers—such as NHL, Hodgkin's disease, soft-tissue and other sarcomas, nasal cancer, nasopharyngeal cancer, and primary hepatic cancer—in Vietnam veterans. Hepatic, nasal-cavity, and nasopharyngeal cancers and Hodgkin's disease were of a priori interest because they had been associated with exposure to phenoxy herbicides, such as Agent Orange, in some animal studies and a few human studies. The 1,157 study participants received a first diagnosis of cancer in 1984–1988 and were listed in any of eight city or state cancer registries—those in Atlanta, Detroit, San Francisco, Seattle, Miami, Connecticut, Iowa, and Kansas. The 1,776 controls were selected by random-digit telephone dialing in the relevant locations and frequency matched by age to the men with cancer. Analyses were adjusted for many demographic, exposure, and medical covariates. Exposure was determined on the basis of characteristics of service in Vietnam, including duration of service and calendar years, age at first tour, rank, unit type, corps (area), and land or sea duty. During the Vietnam War, the military divided South Vietnam into four administrative zones, I–IV Corps; I Corps was the farthest north, and IV Corps was in the southernmost part of the country.

Blue Water Navy veterans had substantially higher risks (OR 2.17, 95% CI 1.22–3.86), including the second-highest risk of NHL in personnel in the various corps (Table 6-2). Only ground troops that served in I Corps had a higher risk of NHL. The authors concluded that the roughly 50% increase in NHL risk in all Vietnam veterans was due to service in Vietnam in general rather than to specific characteristics of service and Agent Orange exposure.

Similarly, for Hodgkin's disease, the highest risk was in I Corps, followed by the Blue Water Navy (OR 1.39, 95% CI 0.56–3.46). There were no cases of Hodgkin's disease in shore-based or Brown Water Navy personnel in this study (Table 6-3).

For soft-tissue and other sarcomas, a decreased risk among Blue Water Navy personnel was observed on the basis of only three cases (OR 0.64, 95% CI 0.18–2.21). For the other cancers tracked in this study, no results were presented for the Blue Water Navy, because there were only two cases of nasal carcinoma, three cases of nasopharyngeal carcinoma, and eight cases of primary hepatic cancer identified for all military service in Vietnam in this study combined.

TABLE 6-2 Association of Selected Characteristics of Military Service in Vietnam with NHL in the Selected Cancers Study, 1984–1988

Characteristic	Controls (n = 1,776)	NHL Cases (n = 1,157)	OR (95% CI)
Corps in Vietnam			
I	18.9% (23)	25.3% (23)	2.25 (1.21–4.18)
II	24.6% (30)	20.9% (19)	1.22 (0.66–2.26)
III	32.8% (40)	20.9% (19)	0.89 (0.50–1.58)
IV	3.3% (4)	2.2% (2)	0.90 (0.15–5.41)
Navy, Blue Water	20.5% (25)	30.8% (28)	2.17 (1.22–3.86)
Unknown	— (11)	— (8)	—
Land v. sea duty in Vietnam			
All land-based men	81.2% (108)	71.7% (71)	1.30 (0.93–1.82)
All branches other than Navy	76.7% (102)	67.7% (67)	1.29 (0.92–1.82)
Navy, shore	3.0% (4)	4.0% (4)	2.26 (0.52–9.78)
Navy, Brown Water	1.5% (2)	— (0)	—
Navy, Blue Water	18.8% (25)	28.3% (28)	2.18 (1.23–3.87)

SOURCE: CDC, 1990a.

Dalager et al.

A hospital-based case–control study examined risks of NHL and Hodgkin's disease in Vietnam veterans or era veterans seen in VA hospitals in 1969–1985 (Dalager et al., 1991, 1995). Study participants were born in 1937–1954. The number of veterans who had NHL was compared with the number of veterans who had diagnoses other than NHL. Exposure was determined on the basis of having served or not having served in Vietnam or on the basis of surrogates of Agent Orange exposure, including branch of service, combat-duty occupation, or corps.

For the investigation of NHL risk, 201 cases and 358 controls were ascertained. Service in Vietnam was not associated with an increased risk of NHL (OR 1.03, 95% CI 0.70–1.50). In Navy veterans ever in Vietnam, the OR was 0.70 (95% CI 0.31–1.60) for NHL. The 283 Hodgkin's disease cases were compared with 404 controls; the result was an OR of 1.28 (95% CI 0.94–1.76) for any service in Vietnam. For the

TABLE 6-3 Association of Selected Characteristics of Military Service in Vietnam with Hodgkin's Disease in the Selected Cancers Study, 1984–1988

Characteristic	Controls (n = 1,776)	Hodgkin's Disease Cases (n = 1,157)	OR (95% CI)
Corps in Vietnam			
I	18.9% (23)	25.9% (7)	1.67 (0.67–4.18)
II	24.6% (30)	11.1% (3)	0.52 (0.15–1.81)
III	32.8% (40)	33.3% (9)	1.25 (0.57–2.75)
IV	3.3% (4)	3.7% (1)	0.93 (0.09–9.82)
Navy, Blue Water	20.5% (25)	25.9% (7)	1.39 (0.56–3.48)
Unknown	— (11)	— (1)	—
Land v. sea duty in Vietnam			
All land-based men	81.2% (108)	75.0% (21)	1.08 (0.64–1.82)
All branches other than Navy	76.7% (102)	75.0% (21)	1.18 (0.70–2.00)
Navy, shore	3.0% (4)	—	—
Navy, Brown Water	1.5% (2)	—	—
Navy, Blue Water	18.8% (25)	25.0% (7)	1.41 (0.57–3.50)

SOURCE: CDC, 1990c.

Navy, the OR was 1.09 (95% CI 0.93–1.28). For both outcomes, neither service in Vietnam in general nor service in the Navy in Vietnam conferred a higher risk. Results were not confounded by age, year of hospitalization, race, or education. Results do not support any association between NHL or Hodgkin's disease and surrogates of Agent Orange exposure in Vietnam veterans.

The use of hospital-ascertained cases and controls may limit the generalizability of results to all Vietnam veterans (those hospitalized are different from other veterans) and introduce bias (exposed cases are more likely to be hospitalized than controls). It was also not possible to determine whether controls were hospitalized for diseases related to service in Vietnam.

OTHER NAVY VETERAN STUDIES

Two studies by Garland et al. (1987, 1988) examined Navy veterans who served during the decade after the end of the Vietnam War. The committee considered this population to be potentially relevant even though they were not Vietnam veterans. The results of the two studies are valuable because they provide background on the potential effects of occupational exposures in Navy personnel who were not in the Vietnam environment; that is, they examined potential occupational exposures other than herbicides.

In a prospective study of cancer incidence, Garland et al. (1987, 1988) examined white male Navy veterans by occupation while they were in service from 1974 to 1979 and compared them with the general US population. It was not a study of Vietnam veterans. Data collected by the Naval Health Research Center included occupational and hospitalization information. Cases of NHL and Hodgkin's disease were identified from hospitalization records and corroborated with medical records or pathologic confirmation.

To assess the risk of Hodgkin's disease, the authors included 2.275 million person-years at risk and 88 cases. The age-adjusted incidence in Navy veterans was 2.9 per 100,000 person-years, lower than the 3.7 per 100,000 person-years reported in the general population (SIR 0.8, 95% CI 0.6–1.0). The average annual age-adjusted incidence in Navy personnel increased with duration of service from 2.3 per 100,000 person-years in those serving less than 2 years to 4.0 per 100,000 person-years for those serving 11 years or more (not statistically significant). After stratification by occupation, a significantly increased risk of Hodgkin's disease was found only in the machinist's-mate occupational category (SIR 2.3, 95% CI 1.2–4.0) compared with a Navy control population. No occupations differed significantly from the US population.

Following the same cohort through 1983, the study included 3.7 million person-years at risk and found 68 cases of NHL. No increased risk of NHL was found; rather, the incidence of NHL in Navy personnel was significantly lower than that in the US population (6.9 versus 9.9 per 100,000 person-years) with an overall SIR of 0.7 (95% CI 0.5–0.9). After stratification by occupation, there were no significant findings, mainly because there were few cases.

Those findings do not indicate an association between NHL or Hodgkin's disease and naval service in the short term. Follow-up may not have been long enough to capture any excess cases, inasmuch as latency may be up to 35 years. Data were available only on active-duty personnel, not on those who may have left the Navy; this might lead to underestimation of disease incidence. The authors noted that the excess of Hodgkin's disease cases in naval machinists may be due to other exposures that could not be assessed in this analysis, including exposures to solvents, cutting and lubricating oils, metal dusts or vapors, Freon, and radiation. The exposure of most concern would be exposure to benzene, which has been linked to NHL.

CONCLUSIONS

The committee was unable to identify published results, other than those discussed in this chapter, of cancer or noncancer health outcomes or mortality in US Blue Water Navy Vietnam veterans that would shed light on disease risks specific to this group. Several epidemiologic studies have measured TCDD concentrations in human tissues, including Vietnam veterans and people living in southern Vietnam. For example, the Air Force (AF) Health Study (AFHS), a cohort study to evaluate adverse health effects of exposure to Agent Orange, included USAF personnel who played an active part in Operation Ranch Hand and additional USAF personnel presumed not exposed. Other studies have looked for TCDD in biological samples from Vietnam veterans, such as blood and semen from Michigan veterans (Schecter et al., 1986), adipose tissue and plasma in Massachusetts veterans (Schecter et al., 1990), and serum in nonexposed Air Force veterans (Pavuk et al., 2005). To the committee's knowledge, no studies assessing TCDD in biological samples of Blue Water Navy veterans are available. The 2008 *VAO* report (IOM, 2009) notes that

> In trying to harvest evidence from a fairly broad spectrum of populations targeted in epidemiologic studies, the VAO committees have factored in results on Vietnam veterans in general on the grounds that they are representative of all subjects who might have had increased exposure to herbicide components (as surrogates for VA's clientele). With respect to the Blue Water Navy issue, the AFHS data document that

> herbicide spraying did not occur solely in Vietnam and did not affect only those deployed to Vietnam. Serum TCDD results from the AFHS demonstrate that the Ranch Hands in general were, indeed, more highly exposed than the Southeast Asia (SEA) veterans, but the SEA veterans had serum TCDD concentrations that tended to exceed background values in the US population.

For Navy veterans as a whole, the Australian cancer-incidence study indicated a significantly higher risk of lung cancer (although the study did not adjust for smoking) and prostatic cancer, both of which are currently recognized as TCDD-related malignancies. A previous IOM committee has concluded that there is limited or suggestive evidence of an association between both cancers and Agent Orange exposure (IOM, 2009). The Australian study found significant associations with melanoma and colon cancer, neither of which has been categorized as TCDD-related by the IOM or the VA. The Australian mortality study corroborated the Australian cancer-incidence findings on lung cancer and melanoma. However, both Australian reports found significantly lower risk of NHL, one of the first cancers associated with Agent Orange exposure by the IOM. One study (Dalager et al., 1991) found neither higher nor lower risk of NHL in Vietnam-era Navy veterans. In contrast, the CDC Selected Cancers Study found a significantly higher prevalence of NHL in Blue Water Navy Vietnam veterans. Finally, in a small study, testicular cancer was associated with service in the Navy (although the Blue Water Navy was not specified) in Vietnam veterans, although testicular cancer has not been found by the IOM to be associated with Agent Orange exposure (IOM, 2009).

There are numerous limitations for this small number of studies. Many did not distinguish between Blue Water Navy and Brown Water Navy populations (or Navy personnel serving on the ground). None characterized exposure to Agent Orange, the committee's primary focus. Some studies are further limited by their small numbers of cases. In addition, some of the studies are hospital-based case–control studies and thus have low generalizability for drawing inferences about risks to the entire Blue Water Navy population. Hospitalization studies typically are conducted in selected hospitals, such as those of the VA or the Department of Defense (DoD), and therefore they are not representative of the entire veteran population, including those no longer on active duty in the case of DoD or veterans who are eligible for but do not seek treatment from the VA. In addition, not all health outcomes require hospitalization, so such cases may not be representative of the entire veteran population.

Confounding factors—such as smoking, alcohol use, and sun exposure—are major contributors to some of the cancers identified as increased in the Australian studies of naval personnel. For example, lung cancer and melanoma were found to be higher in the Australian incidence study. Naval personnel are exposed to some chemicals that have carcinogenic potential, and these were not considered in the analyses of any of the above studies. In the selection of the general male Australian population as a comparison group, the Australian studies did not account for those other exposures and therefore did not account for a healthy-veteran effect. A third report compared Australian Vietnam veterans with era veterans who were stationed in Australia to correct for any healthy-worker effect but did not present results specific to the Navy.

The CDC studies, which showed an increase in NHL, are the most robust, having adjusted for smoking, socioeconomic factors, and a variety of known risk factors for NHL. However, they are the only studies that have identified this link.

Overall, the committee concludes that because of the small number of studies and their limitations, there is no consistent evidence to suggest that Blue Water Navy Vietnam veterans were at higher or lower risk for cancer or other long-term health outcomes than shore-based veterans, Brown Water Navy veterans, or Vietnam veterans in other branches of service.

REFERENCES

Bullman, T. A., K. K. Watanabe, and H. K. Kang. 1994. Risk of testicular cancer associated with surrogate measures of Agent Orange exposure among Vietnam veterans on the Agent Orange Registry. *Annals of Epidemiology* 4(1):11-16.

CDC (Centers for Disease Control and Prevention). 1990a. The association of selected cancer with service in the US military in Vietnam. I. Non-Hodgkin's lymphoma. *Archives of Internal Medicine* 150(12):2473-2483.

CDC. 1990b. The association of selected cancer with service in the US military in Vietnam. II. Soft-tissue and other sarcomas. *Archives of Internal Medicine* 150(12):2485-2492.

CDC. 1990c. The association of selected cancer with service in the US military in Vietnam. III. Hodgkin's disease, nasal cancer, nasopharyngeal cancer, and primary liver cancer. *Archives of Internal Medicine* 150(12):2495-2505.

Dalager, N. A., H. K. Kang, L. B. Burt, and L. Weatherbee. 1991. Non-Hodgkin's lymphoma among Vietnam veterans. *Journal of Occupational Medicine* 33(7):774-779.

Dalager, N. A., H. K. Kang, L. B. Burt, and L. Weatherbee. 1995. Hodgkin's disease and Vietnam service. *Annals of Epidemiology* 5(5):400-406.

Garland, F. C., E. D. Gorham, and C. F. Garland. 1987. Hodgkin's disease in the US Navy. *International Journal of Epidemiology* 16(3):367-372.

Garland, F. C., E. D. Gorham, C. F. Garland, and J. A. Ferns. 1988. Non-Hodgkin's lymphomas in US Navy personnel. *Archives of Environmental Health* 43(2):425-429.

IOM (Institute of Medicine). 2009. *Veterans and Agent Orange: Update 2008*. Washington, DC: The National Academies Press.

Pavuk, M., J. E. Michalek, A. Schecter, N. S. Ketchum, F. Z. Akhtar, and K. A. Fox. 2005. Did TCDD exposure or service in southeast Asia increase the risk of cancer in air force Vietnam veterans who did not spray Agent Orange? *Journal of Occupational and Environmental Medicine* 47(4):335-342.

Schecter, A. J., J. J. Ryan, and J. D. Constable. 1986. Chlorinated dibenzo-p-dioxin and dibenzo-p-furant levels in human adipose-tissue and milk samples from the north and south of Vietnam. *Chemosphere* 15(9-12):1613-1620.

Schecter, A., J. J. Ryan, J. D. Constable, R. Baughman, J. Bangert, P. Furst, K. Wilmers, and R. P. Oates. 1990. Partitioning of 2,3,7,8-chlorinated dibenzo-para-dioxins and dibenzofurans between adipose-tissue and plasma-lipid of 20 Massachusetts Vietnam veterans. *Chemosphere* 20(7-9):951-958.

Wilson, E .J., K. W. Horsley, and R. van der Hoek. 2005a. *Australian National Service Vietnam Veterans Mortality and Cancer Incidence Study 2005*. Canberra, Australia: Department of Veterans' Affairs.

Wilson, E. J., K. W. Horsley, and R. van der Hoek. 2005b. *Australian Vietnam Veterans Mortality Study 2005*. Canberra, Australia: Department of Veterans' Affairs.

Wilson, E. J., K. W. Horsley, and R. van der Hoek. 2005c. *Cancer Incidence in Australian Vietnam Veterans Study 2005*. Canberra, Australia: Department of Veterans' Affairs.

7

SUMMARY AND CONCLUSIONS

The Committee on Blue Water Navy Vietnam Veterans and Agent Orange Exposure was tasked with describing possible mechanisms and routes of exposure of Blue Water Navy personnel to herbicides and their contaminants and comparing the magnitude of their exposure with that of ground troops and Brown Water Navy personnel. Epidemiologic and health-effects data on the herbicides used in Vietnam have been generated primarily on Agent Orange and its toxic contaminant, 2,3,7,8-tetrachlorodibenzo-p-dioxin (TCDD). The Institute of Medicine's (IOM's) *Veterans and Agent Orange* reports have reviewed the health effects data on Agent Orange–associated TCDD and found sufficient evidence of an association between exposure to Agent Orange and five health outcomes (soft-tissue sarcoma, non-Hodgkin's lymphoma, chronic lymphocytic leukemia, Hodgkin's disease, and chloracne). Given the extensive review of the long-term health effects literature by these IOM committees, this committee focused it efforts on determining whether Blue Water Navy veterans had the potential for exposure to Agent Orange–associated TCDD and comparable long-term adverse health risks as their ground troop and Brown Water Navy counterparts.

After considering the many reports on Agent Orange's use and effects in Vietnam—such as the *VAO* series and other IOM reports on Agent Orange (IOM, 2003, 2008)—and other sources of information, such as veterans' accounts of their wartime experiences, the committee decided that the best approach to its tasks was to assess the environmental fate and transport of Agent Orange and TCDD and then to determine whether there were plausible exposure routes by which Blue Water Navy personnel might have come into contact with TCDD during the Vietnam War. The committee also sought to determine whether any information in the literature suggested that Blue Water Navy Vietnam veterans suffered from adverse health effects similar to those of ground troops or troops that served in the military during the war but were not deployed to Vietnam (era veterans).

The committee began with the assumption that it would be possible to determine whether Blue Water Navy personnel were exposed to Agent Orange, how many might have been exposed, and the extent of their exposure. After a review of the available information, the committee decided that it would be necessary to approach its task by evaluating

- Whether it is possible to demonstrate that Blue Water Navy personnel were or were not exposed to Agent Orange–associated TCDD, and
- Whether it is possible to state with certainty that exposure of Blue Water Navy personnel to TCDD, taken as a group, was qualitatively different from that of their Brown Water Navy and ground troop counterparts.

PRIOR EXPOSURE ASSESSMENTS

Since the 1970s, IOM committees and other groups have attempted to determine or reconstruct Vietnam veterans' potential exposure to Agent Orange and TCDD. In particular, two IOM committees assessed an exposure-opportunity model developed by Columbia University principal investigator Jeanne Stellman (IOM, 2003, 2008). The Stellman model is based on the Department of Defense Herbicide Reporting System files on Operation Ranch Hand spraying missions and military personnel records of veterans who served on the ground in Vietnam, including Army, Marine, Navy, and Air Force personnel. The model assigned an exposure-opportunity index value to individuals or groups that had homogeneous exposure characteristics (location and time) that were based on proximity to flight paths of aerial spraying missions and time concordance between spraying and presence in the affected areas. Full application of the exposure-opportunity model to ground troops in Vietnam was never accomplished and has never been proposed for Brown Water Navy or Blue Water Navy personnel.

The suitability of the model for classifying ground troops by degree of probable exposure for the purposes of epidemiologic study has been the subject of some discussion and analysis. The IOM report *The Utility of Proximity-Based Herbicide Exposure Assessment in Epidemiologic Studies of Vietnam Veterans* (IOM, 2008) concluded that the Stellman approach was reasonable, that the model for all its approximations held promise for developing exposure information suitable for epidemiologic studies of Agent Orange health effects, and that the model should be implemented by the Department of Veterans Affairs (VA). The application of the model for units or groups, even with very large-scale distinctions in time or location, has not been attempted. Other investigators have identified diferences in predicted ground-level spray deposition in the Stellman model compared with established pesticide-spray drift models, such as AgDRIFT. The lack of accuracy, precision, and completeness in troop-location data has also been identified as a limitation that would prevent the Stellman approach from being applied reliably to epidemiologic studies (Ginevan et al., 2009a,b). However, alternatives to the Stellman exposure-opportunity model have not been proposed. Concentrations of Agent Orange–associated TCDD in the Vietnamese environment during or shortly after the war or the number of military troops that might have been exposed to Agent Orange–associated TCDD have not been determined.

LIMITATIONS OF AND UNCERTAINTIES IN THE AVAILABLE INFORMATION

Numerous limitations and uncertainties are associated with the information that the committee used to come to its conclusions. Chief among them is the lack of environmental monitoring data on TCDD in Vietnam during the war. The committee relied on previous IOM reports (IOM, 1994, 2003, 2008, 2009) for an assessment of potential exposure of ground troops to TCDD, but those reports did not include exposure assessments for Brown Water Navy or Blue Water Navy personnel. Lack of information on the Brown Water Navy or Blue Water Navy activities, on the use of Agent Orange, and on environmental monitoring contributed to the uncertainties surrounding their potential exposure to TCDD. The committee accepted the conclusions of previous IOM committees that evaluated the utility of the Stellman exposure-opportunity model; however, the value of that model to the present committee's charge was minimal in that no exposure values had been generated.

The committee did not believe that its charge included a review of the VA's current approach to determining whether a Blue Water Navy veteran had been exposed to Agent Orange as that is a policy decision by the VA. The committee notes, however, that for a Blue Water Navy sailor to be eligible for compensation, the sailor or the VA must show that the sailor's ship meets the criteria for classification as a Brown Water Navy vessel during a specified period and that the sailor was aboard the ship at this time. That is a time-consuming task for both the Navy veteran and the VA in that it requires a review of each ship's deck logs.

Finally, the committee spoke with and received information from numerous Vietnam veterans about their war experiences. That information was helpful in providing the committee with an appreciation of the activities of Blue Water Navy personnel (and other veterans) during the war, but some of the information was contradictory, and confirmation of specific events was not possible or was unavailable to the committee. Although records of such events as spray missions were kept, the committee recognizes that events could occur during missions that would alter the flight path of an approved mission (for example, there may have been enemy fire, mechanical problems may have resulted in the spraying of more or less herbicide, and the mission may have been aborted or the herbicide dumped); some such alterations may be recorded, but it is possible that the records are not entirely accurate. The committee greatly appreciated each veteran's input but notes the difficulty in interpreting and using this type of information in assessing population exposure.

The committee notes that Blue Water Navy personnel were also exposed to numerous chemicals during active duty that are known to exert chronic adverse health effects. However, as with TCDD exposure, there were no quantitative measurements of the environmental concentrations of those chemicals aboard US Navy ships during the war. During its tour of the *USS Midway*, the committee noted that Blue Water Navy personnel could have been exposed to a mixture of chemicals on the ships including polychlorinated biphenyls and asbestos, among other hazardous chemicals. Given that a tour of duty was typically 1 year, it is possible that the Navy personnel were exposed to a variety of hazardous chemicals, including chemicals used for occupational purposes, such as solvents and fuels, and those from the ubiquitous cigarette smoke, during the entire period.

Another approach to determining whether Blue Water Navy personnel may have been exposed to TCDD would be to assess the incidence of TCDD-associated adverse health effects in this group of veterans and compare it with the incidence of the same adverse health effects in ground troops and Brown Water Navy personnel. A similar pattern of incidence might be evidence of comparable exposure, and a higher incidence might indicate greater exposure. However, such incidence data are not available on Blue Water Navy personnel. With few exceptions, Blue Water Navy personnel have not been distinguished as a separate cohort in epidemiologic studies of Vietnam veterans. Therefore, the committee was unable to determine, using this approach, whether Blue Water Navy personnel had a greater or smaller potential for exposure to TCDD and for developing adverse health effects. Studies of Royal Australian Navy Vietnam veterans were inconsistent with US studies that associated TCDD exposure with non-Hodgkin's lymphoma. Many of the studies do not account for the high prevalence of cigarette smoking or possible exposure to secondhand smoke aboard naval vessels during the Vietnam War. The conflicting information on the prevalence of non-Hodgkin's lymphoma in Australian versus American Vietnam veterans suggests that further follow-up on the health of the latter population, particularly for Blue Water Navy veterans who had considerable opportunity for exposure to numerous toxic chemicals during their tours of duty, is warranted.

CONCLUSIONS

The committee first approached its task by attempting to estimate the concentrations of TCDD that might have been in the coastal waters of Vietnam as a result of the spraying of Agent Orange during Operation Ranch Hand. This information could then be used to determine possible exposure mechanisms and exposure opportunities of Blue Water Navy personnel. A search of the literature indicated that no measurements of TCDD in any environmental medium in Vietnam had been made during the war or shortly enough after the war to provide reasonable estimates of environmental concentrations. Therefore, the committee explored a modeling approach that used fate and transport considerations in conjunction with multimedia dioxin models developed for other purposes. However, those models are complex and require extensive input data on the Vietnamese environment pertinent to the time of Agent Orange release as well as data on the characteristic behavior of TCDD in that environment. Input parameters are subject to extensive uncertainty, and model results cannot be evaluated for their veracity. Therefore, the committee was not able to estimate even a range of environmental concentrations of TCDD that might be present in Vietnamese coastal waters or the amount of TCDD that might reach Blue Water Navy ships as a result of spray drift from Operation Ranch Hand missions flown near the coast.

With regard to exposure modeling, the committee recognized that despite a substantial investment of time and resources for determining the potential exposure of Vietnam veterans who had served on the ground to Agent Orange–associated TCDD, no actual exposure values have been determined. Nevertheless, the committee did consider whether worst-case scenarios might be helpful in estimating potential exposures for Blue Water Navy veterans. The committee did attempt to do some "back of the envelope" calculations but determined that the uncertainties in the input parameters such as concentrations of TCCD in marine water, ship locations, and dates and locations of spraying missions near the coast, invalidated any exposure estimates. Furthermore, the committee believed that any worst-case estimates might be taken out of context and might be misconstrued as actual exposure estimates. Given the lack of exposure data on ground troops and the knowledge that Brown Water Navy and Blue Water Navy veterans had not even been considered in such exposure-opportunity modeling, the committee concluded that it was not possible to make quantitative exposure comparisons among the three military populations of interest to the VA nor was it possible to do any worst-case bounding of exposure estimates. Therefore, the committee approached the task by evaluating the *plausibility* of exposure of the three populations to Agent Orange and TCDD via various mechanisms and routes.

Even with the lack of quantitative exposure information, the committee recognized that considerable variability exists in the potential for TCDD exposure of Blue Water Navy personnel and ground troops and Brown Water Navy personnel. It is possible that some fraction of Blue Water Navy personnel were not exposed to Agent Orange–associated TCDD, either directly or indirectly, but the proportion of personnel for whom that would have been the case is not known nor is it estimable with available information; there are similar uncertainties in estimating exposure of ground troops and Brown Water Navy sailors and the proportion of those personnel who might have been exposed. Some Blue Water Navy personnel may have spent their entire tour of duty on aircraft carriers that never came close to the Vietnamese coast, and others served on ships (for example, destroyers) that may have spent many days as close as a mile offshore. In addition to the variability in the location of

Blue Water Navy personnel, there is extensive uncertainty regarding the experiences of individual sailors on those ships (for example, whether they were on a ship when it was near the Vietnamese coast, whether they went swimming, and whether they ate local food from Vietnam or Vietnamese waters).

The committee concludes that, qualitatively, ground troops and Brown Water Navy personnel had more pathways of exposure to Agent Orange–associated TCDD than did Blue Water Navy personnel (see Figure 5-1). One exposure mechanism is specific to Blue Water Navy ships: possible TCDD contamination of potable water from shipboard distillation plants. The committee's assessment corroborates the Australian finding that in experiments simulating the water-distillation system used on Navy ships the system had the potential to enrich TCDD concentrations from the feed water to the distilled potable water. However, without information on the TCDD concentrations in the marine feed water, it is impossible to determine whether Blue Water Navy personnel were exposed to TCDD via ingestion, dermal contact, or inhalation of potable water.

After examining a wealth of information on possible routes of exposure, the committee concluded that it would not be possible to determine Agent Orange–associated TCDD concentrations in the Vietnamese environment. This lack of information makes it impossible to quantify exposures for Blue Water and Brown Water Navy sailors and, so far, for ground troops as well. Thus, the committee was unable to state with certainty whether Blue Water Navy personnel were or were not exposed to Agent Orange and its associated TCDD. Moreover, the committee concluded that it could not state with certainty that exposures to Blue Water Navy personnel, taken as a group, were qualitatively different from their Brown Water Navy and ground troop counterparts. Indeed, the committee felt that the paucity of scientific data makes it impossible to determine whether or not Blue Water Navy veterans were exposed to Agent Orange–associated TCDD during the Vietnam War.

REFERENCES

Ginevan, M. E., J. H. Ross, and D. K. Watkins. 2009a. Assessing exposure to allied ground troops in the Vietnam War: A comparison of AgDRIFT and Exposure Opportunity Index models. *Journal of Exposure Science and Environmental Epidemiology* 19(2):187-200.

Ginevan, M. E., D. K. Watkins, J. H. Ross, and R. A. O'Boyle. 2009b. Assessing exposure to allied ground troops in the Vietnam war: A quantitative evaluation of the Stellman Exposure Opportunity Index model. *Chemosphere* 75(11):1512-1518.

IOM (Institute of Medicine). 1994. *Veterans and Agent Orange: Health effects of herbicides used in Vietnam*. Washington, DC: National Academy Press.

IOM. 2003. *Characterizing exposure of veterans to Agent Orange and other herbicides used in Vietnam*. Washington, DC: The National Academies Press.

IOM. 2008. *The utility of proximity-based herbicide exposure assessment in epidemiologic studies of Vietnam veterans*. Washington, DC: The National Academies Press.

IOM. 2009. *Veterans and Agent Orange: Update 2008*. Washington, DC: The National Academies Press.

APPENDIX

CODISTILLATION DURING POTABLE WATER TREATMENT: ANALYSIS OF THE AUSTRALIAN STUDY

Distillation is the oldest method for desalinating marine water for the production of potable water (El-Nashar, 1980). During the 1700s, the US and British navies were making stills from pots; and by the middle 1800s, small stills were being built into shipboard stoves. By the 1940s, all major naval vessels and passenger ships had distillers.

Distillation units were commonly used during World War II to provide sailors with potable water because distillation usually does not require additional chemicals or substantial pretreatment and has relatively low maintenance costs. The committee learned on its site visit to the aircraft carrier, the *USS Midway*, that marine water is taken up and passes through a sieve to remove large debris such as seaweed; the sieve does not remove particulate matter from the marine water. There was no further filtration of marine water before entering the distillation plant. During thermal distillation, a saline solution is heated to generate water vapor, which is then directed to a cool surface, where it can be condensed to liquid water that will contain little salt. Although water boils at 100°C at atmospheric pressure, thermal distillation can be designed to boil water at lower temperatures and at low pressures. At 25% of atmospheric pressure, for example, water will boil at 65°C; at 10% atmospheric pressure, water will boil at 45°C.

The three types of distillation processes are multistage flash (MSF), multiple-effect distillation, and mechanical vapor compression. MSF distillation uses several stages with successively lower temperature and pressure (for example, stage 1: 64°C and 23 inches Hg and stage 2: 46°C and 27 inches Hg (NAVEDTRA 14151)) to rapidly vaporize (flash vaporize) water, which is then condensed by tubes of the inflowing feed water, recovering energy from the heat of condensation. MSF is the most common type of distillation used on ships. The ships typically operate MSF with two- to six-stage flash distillers. The ratio of product water to feed water is about 1 gal of product water per 10–20 gal of feed water. MSF distillation units on Navy surface ships range from 6,000 to 100,000 gal/day (Rankin et al., 1975). Distillation will reject almost all dissolved species, but distillers are sensitive to volatile contaminants that may evaporate from the feed stream. Few or no data exist to verify the contaminant load in the potable water onboard Navy ships; if there is a need to understand the concentration of contaminants in potable water, experiments or models would have to be used to reconstruct the distillation process and offer some clarity.

AUSTRALIAN STUDY

In 2002, researchers at the National Research Centre for Environmental Toxicology (NRCET) and the Queensland Health Scientific Services in Australia conducted a study designed to investigate the potential for exposure of Australian sailors to phenoxy herbicides (such as Agent Orange) contaminated with 2,3,7,8-tetrachlorodibenzo-p-dioxin (TCDD) and dimethylarsinic acid (DMA) through potable water (Muller et al., 2002). The goal of the study, titled "Examination of the Potential Exposure of Royal Australian Navy (RAN) Personnel to Polychlorinated Dibenzodioxins and Polychlorinated Dibenzofurans via Drinking Water" (hereafter the NRCET study), was to determine whether polychlorinated dibenzodioxins (PCDDs) and polychlorinated dibenzofurans (PCDFs) were codistilled during distillation of estuarine waters to produce potable water. Experiments were designed to mimic distillation procedures aboard RAN ships and used a simple rotary evaporator to simulate MSF.

The distillation portion of the study comprised three different stages: (1) reverse osmosis[1] (RO) water spiked with PCDD/Fs (polychlorinated dibenzodioxins and furans; TCDD was spiked at 40 ng/L) and DMA, (2) RO water spiked with contaminants and salt (15 g/L and 30 g/L, respectively), and (3) RO water spiked with total suspended solids (TSS) (0–1.44 g/L TSS). Results were generally presented as percentages of distilled water versus relative retention time of

---

[1]Reverse osmosis is a filtration method that removes many types of large molecules and ions from solution by applying pressure to the solution when it is on one side of a selective membrane.

contaminant (an indirect parameter that is correlated to vapor pressure and solubility). The study concluded that substantial codistillation occurred, especially in the first fraction (14%) of the total starting volume of water distilled. Later aliquots of distilled water contained markedly less contaminant. It should be noted that reverse osmosis was not used aboard US Navy ships during the Vietnam War.

The study showed that there may be some codistillation of semi-volatile contaminants during distillation. If the purpose of this experiment was to demonstrate the plausibility of TCDD exposure to sailors via distilled water, then this study is useful; however, the application of these findings to actual shipboard distillation systems requires knowledge of several factors not addressed in the experiment. The significance of this study's findings for contaminant exposures on Blue Water Navy ships is highly uncertain. Therefore, an independent analysis was conducted in order to determine the likelihood of codistillation of TCDD; this analysis was conducted using a theoretical model.

BATCH DISTILLATION MODELING TO SIMULATE THE AUSTRALIAN STUDY EXPERIMENTAL DATA

The committee considered an equilibrium vaporization process in which the entire feed liquid is charged to the still pot and heat is added continuously. Vapor is continuously produced and removed from the well-mixed vessel. In this batch mode of operation, the liquid product is removed at the end of the run. The operation is often called Rayleigh or batch distillation.

Simulating the NRCET Study

The batch distillation experiment was simulated by solving physical and thermodynamic equations using conditions identical to those of the NRCET study experiments and TCDD as the contaminant. Details of the equations follow. The parameters needed for the calculations based on the conditions of the experiments are as follows:

- Initial TCDD concentration: 40 ng/L (or initial mole fraction, $x_D = 1.242 \times 10^{-12}$).
- Initial amount of feed, L_0: 1 kg (1 L).

- Final amount of feed, L: 0.9 kg (10% of water is distilled).
- Temperature of distillation: 58°C (331 K).
- Dimensionless (mole:volume ratio) Henry constant for TCDD at 25°C (298 K): $K_D^* = 10^{-2.46}$ (Aberg et al., 2008).
- Relative volatility of TCDD at 25°C (298 K): $K_D = 34.1$.
- Relative volatility of TCDD at 58°C (331 K): $K_D = 34.1 \times 23.16 = 789.7$.

Using those parameters, the fraction (and thus the percentage) of TCDD that was codistilled can be calculated. The calculations reveal 100% codistillation of TCDD into 0.1 L of distillate. Therefore, the concentration of TCDD in the distillate is 400 ng/L (40/0.1). That result is in general agreement with the experimental results reported in the NRCET study (75–95% codistillation). The model simulations indicate that TCDD is readily codistilled and thus will be present in the product water of distillation systems using water that contains TCDD. In the section below the committee presents the thermodynamic equations that support this conclusion.

Thermodynamic Basis of Distillation Model

For a binary mixture of species i and j, mass-balance analysis yields the following equation for batch distillation (King, 1980; Wankat, 1988):

$$\ln \frac{L}{L_0} = \int_{x_{i0}}^{x_i} \frac{dx_i}{y_i - x_i} \tag{1}$$

Here, L_0 and x_{i0} are the initial moles of liquid feed to the still pot and the mole fraction of species i in the initial feed, L and x_i are the remaining moles of liquid and mole fraction of species i in the liquid at any time, and y_i is the mole fraction of species i in the vapor phase. To use the equation, it is necessary to have a relationship between y_i and x_i. In the case of batch distillation, an equilibrium relationship between the vapor and liquid phases should be used.

For equilibrium separation processes involving a vapor–liquid system, it is common to use an inherent separation factor termed the relative volatility, which for a binary mixture is defined as

$$\alpha_{ij} = \frac{y_i / x_i}{y_j / x_j} = \frac{K_i}{K_j} \tag{2}$$

where y_i are x_i are the mole fractions of species i in the vapor and liquid phases, y_j and x_j are the mole fractions of species j in the vapor and liquid phases, and K_i and K_j are the corresponding distribution coefficients of species i and j. Because $y_j = 1 - y_i$ and $x_j = 1 - x_i$, Equation 2 represents a relationship between y_i and x_i that can be used in Equation 1.

The relative volatility α_{ij} can be assumed constant; hence, substituting the relationship between y_i and x_i (Equation 2) in Equation 1 yields (King, 1980; Wankat, 1988)

$$\ln\frac{L}{L_0} = \frac{1}{\alpha_{ij}-1}\ln\frac{x_i\left(1-x_{i0}\right)}{x_{i0}\left(1-x_i\right)} + \ln\frac{1-x_{i0}}{1-x_i} \tag{3}$$

For the specific problem at hand of water (W) containing a dioxin congener (D), Equation 3 can be written as

$$\ln\frac{L}{L_0} = \frac{1}{\alpha_{DW}-1}\ln\frac{x_D\left(1-x_{D0}\right)}{x_{D0}\left(1-x_D\right)} + \ln\frac{1-x_{D0}}{1-x_D} \tag{4}$$

Because the water contains a minute amount of TCDD—that is, x_D <<1—Equation 4 simplifies to

$$\ln\frac{L}{L_0} = \frac{1}{\alpha_{DW}-1}\ln\frac{x_D}{x_{D0}} \tag{5}$$

Equation 5 allows us to express the mole fraction of TCDD in the still pot, x_D, as a function of the amount of liquid remaining in the still pot, L:

$$\ln\frac{x_D}{x_{D0}} = \left(\alpha_{DW}-1\right)\ln\frac{L}{L_0} \tag{6}$$

Once x_D is determined by Equation 6, we can find the fraction of TCDD that was codistilled (that is, ended up in the product water) from

$$F = \frac{x_{D0}L_0 - x_D L}{x_{D0}L_0} \tag{7}$$

By using Equation 2, the relative volatility, α_{DW}, can be expressed as the ratio of the distribution coefficients of dioxin and water between the liquid and vapor phases:

$$\alpha_{DW} = \frac{y_D / x_D}{y_W / x_W} = \frac{K_D}{K_W} \tag{8}$$

Because of the very high mole fraction of water in the liquid and the absence of appreciable quantities of inert substances in the vapor, both y_W and x_W are near 1.00, and $K_W \approx 1$. Hence, $\alpha_{DW} = K_D$.

The distribution coefficient of TCDD in water, K_D, can be determined from the dimensionless Henry constant for TCDD, K_D^*, which is based on the ratio of mole:volume concentrations (Aberg et al., 2008). Converting the units of mole fractions in the vapor phase, y_D, and the liquid (water) phase, x_D, to mole:volume concentrations, and rearranging, yields

$$K_D = \frac{y_D}{x_D} = \frac{RT}{PV_w} K_D^* \qquad (9)$$

where R is the gas constant, T the absolute temperature, P the pressure in the distillation pot, and V_w the molar volume of water.

The distribution coefficient or Henry constant for TCDD at 58°C (331 K) is not readily available in the literature. However, the Clausius–Clapeyron relation can be used to determine the Henry constant at 58°C (Aberg et al., 2008):

$$\ln \frac{K_D(T_2)}{K_D(T_1)} = -\frac{\Delta U_D}{R}\left(\frac{1}{T_2} - \frac{1}{T_1}\right) \qquad (10)$$

where $K_D(T_1)$ is the Henry constant at 25°C (known), $K_D(T_2)$ is the Henry constant at 58°C, R is the gas constant, and ΔU_D is the internal energy of phase change for $K_D(T_1)$. The latter can be found in Aberg et al. (2008): $\Delta U_D = 78{,}097$ J/mol. Using that relationship, we find the ratio

$$\frac{K_D(331\ \mathrm{K})}{K_D(298\ \mathrm{K})} = 23.16 \qquad (11)$$

Equations 1–10 were solved using physical properties of TCDD in order to determine the percent of total TCDD in the feed water subject to codistillation. Thus, in the batch distillation process used in the NRCET study (Muller, 2002), a concentration of 40 ng TCDD/L in 1 L feed water would result in all 40 ng TCDD being distilled into the 0.1 L of product water, assuming 10% of the feed water is distilled. This demonstrates an enrichment of TCDD from the feed water into the product water with a product water concentration of 40 ng/0.1 L or 400 ng/L.

REFERENCES

Aberg, A., M. MacLeod, and K. Wiberg. 2008. Physical-chemical property data for dibenzo-p-dioxin (DD), dibenzofuran (DF), and chlorinated DD/Fs: A critical review and recommended values. *Journal of Physical and Chemical Reference Data* 37(4):1997-2008.

El-Nashar, A. M., I. Nusbaum, O. K. Buros, R. Bakish, and R. B. Cox. 1980. *The U.S.A.I.D. desalination manual*. Gainesville, FL: CH2M Hill International Corporation.

King, C. J. 1980. *Separation processes*. Columbus, OH: McGraw-Hill.

Muller, J. F., C. Gaus, K. Bundred, V. Alberts, M. R. Moore, and K. Horsley. 2002. *Examination of the potential exposure of Royal Australian Navy (RAN) personnel to polychlorinated dibenzodioxins and polychlorinated dibenzofurans via drinking water. A report to: The Department of Veteran Affairs, Australia*. Brisbane, Australia: National Research Centre for Environmental Toxicology.

Rankin, B. H., W. B. Huckenpoehler, and W. L. Adamson. 1975. *Investigation of shipboard distilling plant energy consumption*. Bethesda, MD: Department of the Navy, Naval Research and Development Center.

Wankat, P. C. 1988. *Equilibrium stages separations*. Englewood Cliffs: Prentice-Hall.